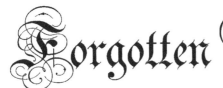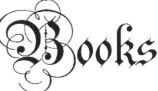
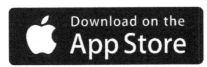
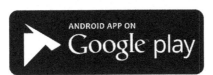

ISBN 978-1-330-14848-8
PIBN 10037788

This book is a reproduction of an important historical work. Forgotten Books uses state-of-the-art technology to digitally reconstruct the work, preserving the original format whilst repairing imperfections present in the aged copy. In rare cases, an imperfection in the original, such as a blemish or missing page, may be replicated in our edition. We do, however, repair the vast majority of imperfections successfully; any imperfections that remain are intentionally left to preserve the state of such historical works.

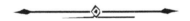

English
Français
Deutsche
Italiano
Español
Português

www.forgottenbooks.com

Mythology Photography **Fiction**
Fishing Christianity **Art** Cooking
Essays Buddhism Freemasonry
Medicine **Biology** Music **Ancient**
Egypt Evolution Carpentry Physics
Dance Geology **Mathematics** Fitness
Shakespeare **Folklore** Yoga Marketing
Confidence Immortality Biographies
Poetry **Psychology** Witchcraft
Electronics Chemistry History **Law**
Accounting **Philosophy** Anthropology
Alchemy Drama Quantum Mechanics
Atheism Sexual Health **Ancient History**
Entrepreneurship Languages Sport
Paleontology Needlework Islam
Metaphysics Investment Archaeology
Parenting Statistics Criminology
Motivational

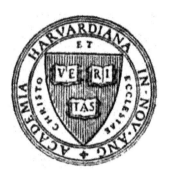

THE VIRILE·POWERS
OF SUPERB MANHOOD

HOW DEVELOPED,
HOW LOST: HOW REGAINED

❦❦❦

By BERNARR A. MACFADDEN
Editor of "Physical Culture,"
(With the assistance of Medical and Other Authorities)

❦❦❦

❦❦❦

PUBLISHED BY THE
PHYSICAL CULTURE PUBLISHING COMPANY
Townsend Building, 25th St. & Broadway
NEW YORK, U. S. A.

To assist in stifling that horrible
curse of prudishness and the ignorance of sex which it entails is the
object which has influenced the writing of this book.

To all those whose souls and bodies are tortured with weakness because of the criminal neglect of prudish parents, or because of their own indiscretions or excesses resulting from ignorance of sex, this book is most respectfully dedicated.

Do not be satisfied with mediocrity: Push onward and upward. If you are not strong, if you have not the energy, the ambition, the power, which lead one above the prosaic, the commonplace, develop it now. Make up your mind that strength and health of a high degree shall be yours, and work for this end with determination and persistence, and superb physical powers will be your glorious reward.

PREFACE.

Numerous books have been written on the subject treated herein, but no one gives sufficient practical knowledge to enable the average reader to apply the necessary treatment required in his own case.

The writer has endeavored to supply this need. He has purposely refrained from all technical phrases, and the contents have been abbreviated as much as possible.

It is the writer's desire to furnish the greatest amount of information in the fewest possible words. He is of the opinion that there are thousands, and perhaps millions, of boys, young men, and even old men, whose powers, mental, physical and sexual, are fast declining because of the need of knowledge which can be supplied here, and he firmly and honestly believes that the contents of this work will do more to elevate, ennoble and strengthen its readers than any other influence of a similar character. It will help them to be *men*—strong, virile, superb—and the first duty of every male human adult is to be a man. All other requirements should be subordinate to this. You cannot build a house without a foundation to rest upon, and virile manhood is the foundation upon which must rest all the results that accrue from education and the refining influences of civilized life. In other words, if you do not possess this virile manhood your imperative duty is to strive for its acquirement, even if necessary for the time being to sacrifice every other purpose in life. For if you are not a man, you are nothing but a nonentity! A cipher! And as long as you remain in this emasculated condition, your powers and capacities in every way will be bound by your weakened condition.

The writer has pointed out the way to acquire and retain these much desired powers. It lies with you. Is the reward a sufficient recompense? If so, begin the work prescribed here at once, for he is no miracle worker. He does not offer you powers, worth more than all the money in the universe, in a few dollars' worth of powders or pills. You must work for such rewards. There is nothing on earth of real value which is acquired without labor, and the powers of manhood are no exception to this rule. You must bring about your own cure.

If there are any who feel that their particular cases are not fully covered, a special course will be prescribed; but please remember that it has taken the writer from four to five times as long to acquire his present knowledge along this line than is required for the average physician to graduate, so for a short letter of advice we shall expect a fee of $2.00, and for a complete course especially outlined for individual needs, a fee of $5.00. Those who desire the $5.00 course, can have a personal interview or examination, or there will be sent them a long question blank to be filled out that their exact physical condition, habits, etc., may be ascertained.

The writer desires to say in conclusion, however, that if this book is carefully studied there should be absolutely no need of special advice. He has found, usually, that those who desire special advice, simply wish to avoid the study necessary in forming accurate conclusions as to the proper treatment in their cases. Therefore, if you desire the writer to do your studying you must expect to pay for it. He has endeavored to meet every possible contingency that will appear in ordinary cases, and though he is aware that everyone is usually under the impression that his case is far from agreeing with the ordinary, still careful study will usually reveal no features essentially different.

The writer does not want your money. He can use his time to better advantage, both financially and otherwise, than in answering your queries. He would rather you would study up your own case and thus be able to answer your own questions, and will candidly state that it will be to your advantage in the end to do this, because you will be following conclusions that are the product of your own reasoning, and if they are wrong the results will soon show it, and then if puzzled you can come to him to solve your problems.

BERNARR A. MACFADDEN.

CONTENTS.

CONTENTS.

CHAPTER I.

THE IMPORTANCE OF VIRILE MANHOOD.

WHERE KNOWLEDGE BECOMES A CURSE.

Man, the king of all animals, still grovels in the dust and mire of ignorance, and even his own boasted knowledge often turns and bites, and stings and enervates, and at times even destroys him. Knowledge of evil without the antidote of knowing its vile and destructive influence, is a condition where knowledge becomes a curse. Knowledge of the momentary pleasures which can be obtained by sexual indulgences, without the knowledge of their terrible deleterious influence under certain unnatural conditions, is one of the greatest causes of physical weakness, and the pain, unhappiness and disease that accompany this abnormal condition.

The sexual power of a man indicates with marvelous accuracy his general physical and mental condition. It is the barometer of the physical and nervous organism.

INTENSE ENTHUSIASM INSPIRED BY VIRILE POWERS.

The fiery ardor of a patriot, the intense ambition of an enthusiast, the inspiration that influences noble deeds of valor, the sacrificial spirit that has time and time again caused the world to ring with praises of some hero, all spring from the same nervous energy which supplies the power of sex,·the power of manhood.

Name any man famous in the world of literature, of art, or of science, and in nearly every instance he will be found to possess evidence of strong virility. The nervous energy, so necessary to the enormous labor which brought his success, was the same power that controlled his sexual instinct.

"Sexuality has been strongly marked in all the great men who have risen to eminence in all departments of life; without it man would be mean, selfish, sordid and ungracious to his fellowmen and uncivil to womankind. Were it not for this nature which God has implanted in our being, no man would desire to provide for the support of another individual, or enter into a relation which would likely impose upon him the necessity of supporting a family of dependent and grow-ing children. No man becomes affable, gracious and considerate to women until he is renderd so by the awakening of his sexual nature and the quickening of that within him, which, when held under proper disci-pline and control, renders him noble and unselfish."—*Sylvanus Stall, D.D.*

CLOSE RELATIONSHIP OF SEXUAL AND PHYSI-CAL HEALTH.

The great importance of strong sexual powers cannot be too strongly emphasized. Their influence on life is marvelous. If a fine, vigorous man acquires a complaint that weakens his sexual organs, his powers in every way will begin to decline—his muscles will grow weaker, his nerves will be affected, and unless a change is quickly made, he will soon become a physical wreck. The nervous, sexual, muscular and vital forces are so closely interwoven that what affects one always influences the others in a similar manner. As the muscles are developed and strengthened the nervous and other powers are favorably influenced if wisely used

The nervous forces depend upon a normal circulation of the blood for their sustenance. Muscular exercise of some kind is absolutely necessary to functional activity of the entire circulatory system.

The mental influence of a strong sexual instinct is seen in all male animals as well as man. It elevates, thrills one with energy, with powers, and no one can for an instant question the conclusion that strength in this way gives a man more power in every walk of life.

PERFECT SEXUAL POWERS GIVEN ONLY TO THE BEST.

It is one of Nature's unfailing laws that the best of her species shall possess the greatest powers of transmitting their kind; and who can for one instant question the conclusion that vigorous sexual powers, temperately and legitimately used, actually brighten and strengthen a man's every faculty, elevate and inspire his every ambition, giving him greater influence and capacity for anything he may attempt in life? But few men by their own efforts have ever accomplished anything of value in life who were not gifted also with a strong sexual instinct.

SEXUAL POWER INDICATES CAPACITY.

The importance of retaining the sexual power, of using it wisely and temperately, cannot be over-estimated. It is paramount. Lose your sexual power, lose the power to reproduce your species, and, according to the laws of nature, your days of usefulness are past, and decay and death will soon over-take you.

Impotence sexually means impotence in everything, impotence mentally, physically, socially, etc. Your powers are fast waning —you might just as well be laid away without further notice.

CHAPTER II.

CAUSES OF LOSS OF MANHOOD.

IGNORANCE AND PRUDISHNESS PRIMARY CAUSES.

The causes are various, but unquestionably the great primary causes are ignorance and the prudishness which it engenders.

Ignorance of the facts in reference to the sexual instinct that should be as plain as the noonday sun to every human being, this, together with lack of knowledge of the great laws of health, so necessary in order to build vigor and symmetry of body, have resulted in filling civilized countries with a host of pigmy men. Immediately after birth they come in contact with abnormal influences. They are encumbered with clothing that discourages rather than encourages muscular movements, they are compelled to breathe foul air when the weather is cold; they are always overfed; the bottle often does duty for the female breast, and they come in contact with all sorts of conditions that tend to depreciate vitality. Of course over half are killed by all this, and those that survive are greatly weakened,. and never attain the superb manhood that should be their inalienable right.

ABNORMAL CONDITIONS THAT CONFRONT ALL BOYS.

From the ages of six to fourteen years, the disgusting and depraved secrecy maintained in all sexual subjects arouses a boy's curiosity, and he finally discovers through evil companions, or by accident, that horrible curse, MASTURBATION. Vitality may have struggled for the mastery before, but now it has an enemy with which it literally has no chance. (See chapter on Masturbation.) When a boy finally escapes from the clutches of this Gorgon evil—though many never escape—he finds that he is cursed with night losses that seem to waste his vitality almost as speedily as the previous evil. (See chapter on Night Losses and Other Drains upon Vital Powers.) He usually escapes from this with his life, and then is confronted with promiscuous intercourse, as practiced almost universally among young men in all civilized countries. (See chapter on Promiscuous Intercourse.) This habit is not practiced long without severe suffering. Some one of the diseases which is the terrible penalty for this plain infraction of Nature's laws is sure to be contracted. Then the torture of body and of mind is terrible. Visions of complete loss of manhood confront him. He may have had dreams of a home, surrounded by a loving wife, and happy, beautiful children. He realizes with stinging keenness the fact that these diseases may forever destroy the possibility of the realization of this beautiful dream. (See chapter on these diseases.) Though many fall by the wayside, the majority get through these last-named contaminating conditions with enough vital and sexual strength to look with favor on marriage.

UNNATURAL MARITAL CONDITIONS.

The girl that such a man marries is usually weak and possesses but little instinct of sex, and then sexual excess begins its frightful ravages on the physical man. (See chapter on Sexual Excess.)

This sexual excess continues usually until impotence intervenes.

There you have the life of the average civilized man !

Think you this picture overdrawn ?

Think you that this is civilization ?

My friends, it is savagery of the lowest, the most bestial character. As long as such a state of affairs exists, we have no more right to the claim of civilization than had those effeminate, corrupt and well-fed patricians of Ancient Rome whose weakness finally resulted in the downfall of that grand empire.

ARE WE, TOO, CONSIGNED TO SPEEDY OBLIVION?

The decay and death of this great people convey a lesson that can not be mistaken, and the writer maintains with all possible emphasis that either existing conditions will soon be changed or else the civilization of which we boast will meet with swift and certain oblivion.

Think you there is no truth in this statement? Let the future answer!

But cry out the truth on the housetops !

A drunkard begins by taking an occasional dram which seems of no importance.

All the vast category of evils enumerated here are really made possible by that Gorgon horror, Masturbation. The most damnable crime ever committed is the neglect of parents to warn their children of this evil which degrades and demoralizes the physical and sexual system, and makes all the terrible evils that follow so easily acquired.

But why go further? Let us pass on to the next chapter and learn more of this horrible curse.

Chapter III.

MASTURBATION.

RESULTS IN FRIGHTFUL LOSS OF MANLY POWERS.

The loss of physical manhood resulting from this one evil is horrible to contemplate. The laws of sex should be as plain as the alphabet to every human being, even from early childhood. Boys grow up without a word said to them on this important subject. They come in contact with the most horrible and most destructive evils of life almost before the real struggle of life begins. They enter it without a word of warning.

This is the usual condition. Think of it, reader. Parents who claim to love their children, allow this.

TERRIBLE ARRAIGNMENT OF THIS EVIL BY AN AUTHORITY.

"Masturbation outrages nature's sexual ordinances more than any or all the other orms of sexual sin man can perpetrate,

and inflicts consequences the most terrible.
It is man's sin of sins, and vice of vices;
and has caused incomparably more sexual
dilapidation, paralysis, and disease, as well
as demoralization, than all the other sexual
depravities combined. Neither Christendom
nor heathendom suffers any evil at all to
compare with this; because of its universal-
ity, and its terrible fatal ravages on body
and mind; and because it attacks the young
idols of our hearts, and hopes of our future
years. Pile all other evils together—drunk-
enness upon all cheateries, swindlings, rob-
beries, and murders; and tobacco upon both,
for it is the greatest scourge; and all sickness, diseases and pestilences upon all; and
war as the cap sheaf of them all—and all
combined cause not a tithe as much human
deterioration and misery as does this secret
sin."—*Prof. O. S. Fowler.*

HANDSOME BOYS WRECKED.

You see a strong, handsome boy, clear-eyed
with beautifully-tinted complexion, straight,
well-formed limbs. You admire his elastic

step, his manly carriage, his fine, wholesome, symmetrically-formed body.

A year or two, or even a few months, intervene, and this boy has learned, through evil associates, or by accident, this secret vice. You see him again, and you may well start with pain and surprise at the change.

Is this the same boy I admired so much? you may exclaim.

There is no light of health in his eyes now; there is no symmetry to his ungainly body, no tint to his sallow cheeks, no grace, or manliness in his bearing. He looks old and weak, appears bashful and timid, seems afraid of your glance. The dark circles under his eyes, unshapely appearance of his lower limbs, and general decrepit and demoralized condition tell a tale that no language can fittingly depict,—the awful results of masturbation.

IGNORANCE THE CAUSE.

"The most fruitful source of self-pollution is ignorance. If parents were faithful in the discharge of their duty to their children in this respect, the evil would be generally corrected. The silence of most parents is both foolish and culpable. The person who leaves his or her child to learn from vicious companions in an unhallowed way what they should have received from the lips of father or mother is guilty of grave neglect, and loses the best opportunity of a parent's life to establish the mind of the child in purity and virtue."—*Sylvanus Stall, D. D.*

Mrs. Alice Lee Moque, herself the mother of three boys, in writing upon this subject aptly and correctly says:

"Ignorance is a dreadful sin. In this enlightened age we must recognize that ignorance is not innocence, and remember that to forewarn our boys is to forearm them. The truth, properly told, has never yet harmed a child; silence, false shame and mystery have corrupted the souls and bodies of untold millions."

YOU CAN'T WARN YOUR BOYS TOO SOON.

"Rendered childless by my husband's ignorance of these private truths you teach, I adopted three sons, whom I determined, by forewarning, to save from this vice, and warned my eldest on his sixteenth birthday;

but was too late, as he owned he had perpetrated it for years. Determined to be in ample season with my other two, I warned my next youngest at thirteen, never dreaming that it could be practiced before puberty; but found myself again too late. Half frantic with disappointment, and determined to make sure of saving my now only undefiled, I warned him at ten; but, horrible to relate was still too late; for he had already learned and perpetrated it!"—*The Founder of the College at Cleveland*.

IT BENUMBS THE BRAIN, NERVES, AND MIND

"The sin of self-pollution is one of the most destructive evils ever practiced by fallen man. In many respects it is several degrees worse than common whoredom, and leaves in its train more awful consequences. It excites the powers of nature to undue action, and produces violent secretions, which necessarily and speedily exhaust the vital principle and energy; hence the muscles become flaccid and feeble, the tone and natural action of the nerves relaxed and impeded, the understanding confused, the memory oblivious, the judgment perverted, the will indeterminate and wholly without energy to resist; the eyes appear languishing and without expression, and the countenance vacant; appetite ceases, for the stomach is incapable of performing its proper office; nutrition fails; tremors, fears, and terrors are generated; and thus the wretched victim drags out a miserable existence, till, super-annuated, even before he had time to arrive at man's estate, with a mind often debili-tated even to a state of idiotism, his worth-less body tumbles into the grave, and his guilty soul (guilty of self-murder) is hurried into the awful presence of its Judge!"— *Adam Clarke's Com. on Onan.*

A PHYSICIAN'S PLAIN WORDS.

"These results of masturbation I have seen in my own practice—involuntary emis-sions, prostration of strength, paralysis of the limbs, hysteria, epilepsy, strange nervous affections, dyspepsia, hypochondria, spinal disease, pain and weakness in the back and limbs, costiveness, and, in fine, the long and dismal array of gastric, enteric, nervous and spinal affections, which are so complicated and difficult to manage."—*Dr. J. A. Brown.*

WEAKNESSES AFTER PUBERTY CAUSED BY IT.

"Many of the ills which come upon the young at and after puberty arise from this habit, persisted in so as to waste their vital energies, and enervate their physical and mental powers. Nature designs that this drain should be reserved until mature age, and even then be made but sparingly. Sturdy manhood, in all its vigor, loses its energy, and bends under the too frequent expenditure of this important secretion; and no age or condition will protect a man from the danger of unlimited indulgence, though legally and naturally exercised.

"In the young, however, its influence is much more seriously felt; and even those who have indulged so cautiously as not to break down their health or minds, cannot know how much their physical energy, mental vigor, and moral purity have been weakened by this indulgence. No cause produces as much insanity. The records of the institutions give an appalling catalogue of cases attributed to it."—*Dr. Woodward.*

THE WORST OF ALL EVILS.

Prostitution and intemperance may do much to demoralize and destroy the character and physique of young men, but unquestionably at the present day, masturbation causes more physical deterioration, more insanity, more tendency to crime, than any other one evil of this character. It takes boys when they are maturing, when the slightest influence effects them, we might say all through life, and literally vulgarizes, degrades and demoralizes them physically, mentally and sexually.

This terrible crime to civilization, to humanity, now being committed by the parents and teachers who ignore these subjects with such studied significance, cannot be too strongly condemned.

ARE WE REALLY CIVILIZED?

No nation has the slightest claim to true civilization when such crimes are daily and hourly perpetrated, without even the slightest effort being made to stop the terrible slaughter of innocents that results from this most base, this most criminal neglect.

What would you think of a man who would unfeelingly stand by a blind child and see it walk to the brink of a precipice and fall into the depth below? Where is the difference between this inhuman creature and a parent or guardian who will stand by and see his child innocently, blindly falling into the abyss of masturbation, which, though it may not mean death, in every case means that the victim will be maimed mentally, morally and physically for life? Of course he often recovers and becomes a good and useful citizen, but he would have been better and stronger and nobler if not tainted and wrecked by such vile influences.

HARSH NAMES FOR PARENTS.

There is no name too harsh with which one could designate such unfeeling, despicable, prudish parents. The lowest animals of the earth protect their own progeny from destructive influences, but these creatures, dressed in clothes that hide their filthy bodies and depraved brains, allow their children to enter these vile pit-falls without a word of protest. If such prudes ever generated an original idea, if there has ever been a single occasion when humanity has been improved, either individually or collectively, because of their having lived, the writer would like to hear of it.

PARENTS WITHOUT HEARTS.

If you are a parent, a guardian, and have one atom of truth, of honor, of love in your heart, warn your *boys*—and your girls, too—of the terrible evils that they must avoid.

Neglect this imperative duty, and if there is *Hell* in the other world, you fully deserve an important position there, for you have assisted in no small way to make a hell on this earth for your own child.

CRIMES OF PARENTS.

There is no crime more dastardly, that deserves more punishment, than this. Adults have some protection against crime. They are fully aware of its existence, but children look up to and depend on their parents for protection, and it would injure them far less if they were beaten on the head near unto death with a club than it would to allow them innocently to acquire and practice this secret vice.

CAUSES MORE MISERY THAN ALL OTHER SEXUAL SINS.

" Private fornication causes twenty times more misery than any other sexual sin. And this is substantially the opinion of all who have examined this subject. If a loved child must practice either—O merciful God! deliver all from such a dilemma—almost as soon let it DIE. Any other cup of bitterness is less bitter! Nothing, O fond parent, can render your beloved offspring more completely wretched."—*Prof. O. S. Fowler.*

IS THERE HOPE FOR THE FALLEN?

Again and again the question is asked, " Can the effect of this terrible evil be eradicated?" A boy can never be the man he might have been had the habit never been practiced, though he can undoubtedly recover from its effects and develop a fine vigorous physique if proper efforts are made. To such an unfortunate the writer would say: Follow the system of exercises illustrated here. Take up all sorts of outdoor exercises. Live in the open air as much as you can, and vow with an unflinching determination that you will be a man—that you will conquer the terrible habit.

Read carefully all the advice in reference to building sexual vigor, and you can depend on complete recovery, and upon the acquirement of a degree of health and strength that will be far above the average, though if the habit has been practiced very long a certain amount of vital and general physical vigor has no doubt been sacrificed beyond recall.

CHAPTER IV.

SEXUAL EXCESS.

ENERVATING EFFECTS.

Many men appear to think and act as though their sexual powers were limitless. Week after week, month after month, and often year after year, they indulge in this way to the extreme limit. The ultimate result is always serious. The body is like a chain which is as strong as its weakest link, and when excess of this character becomes continuous the general vigor is gradually undermined. The muscles lose some of their elasticity, firmness and symmetry; the various vital organs—stomach. heart, lungs —become gradually weaker, and if there is any physical defect or a tendency towards any disease, the general weakened condition of the body enables it easily to develop. Thousands of men have died and are still dying of consumption and other wasting diseases which are made possible because of the weakness brought about through sexual excess.

PROCREATION THE AIM OF INTERCOURSE.

" In nature, sexual intercourse has but one aim, and that is procreation. This act, which is one of the greatest mysteries of life, and should be reverenced as a sacrament, should be performed only for the purpose of securing offspring. Every other such act, or sexual excitement, constitutes vice, undermines health, and is a sacrilege against Nature's laws ordained by God Almighty. For the purpose of procreation, one act may suffice; then, while the fruit is developing, and also during the time of nursing, the mother should abstain. This state of affairs we find with all wild animals."—*A. F. Reinhold, Ph. D., M. D.*

RICHNESS OF THIS VITAL FLUID.

Excess in this way seems to destroy the energies, takes away the ambition. Some physiologists claim that one drop of the semen is equal to sixty drops of blood. Although it would unquestionably be difficult to determine accurately the relative value of this vital fluid compared to the blood, no one will question its richness in vital elements. It contains the very essence of a man, for is it not bone of his bone, flesh of his flesh?

The especial fact to be deplored in connection with this character of intemperance is that many do not appear to be aware of its deleterious effects.

They begin to decline when addicted to excess, and blame it on a cold accidentally acquired, or to other senseless causes which in no way assisted in bringing about their condition.

MARRY A REAL WOMAN—NOT A WRECK.

While writing along this line it would be well to mention the enormous importance of marrying a girl who has sufficient stamina to be normal in this way. Many women, because of their weakened and general abnormal condition, are void of all instinct, so important in protecting themselves and their husbands from these excesses. In every normal healthy woman there are periods when these intimate relations are repugnant,

and Nature created these periods as a protection against these excesses. (See chapter on
Why Marriage sometimes Wrecks.)

Though deplorable, it is nevertheless a
fact that because of the unnatural conditions,
corsets, long shirts, etc., etc., which contami-
nate and deteriorate the bodies of growing
girls, but few of them grow into normal
womanhood, possessors of the superfine instinct so necessary for their own and their
life-partner's protection against such serious
excesses.

LAMENTABLE RESULTS OF MARRYING INVALIDS TO-BE.

"At times, while under the infatuation and
blinding influences of courtship, a young
man who fully realizes the physical infirmities of the young woman with whom he is
keeping company, will excuse all her aches
and ills, and, under the delusion that it will
be a pleasure to nurse her in her sickness
and minister to her many infirmities, deliber-
ately decide upon marriage. If you are in
love with such a young woman, you cannot
possibly be more cruel to her than to marry
her. Let her condition appeal to your mercy,

and if you love her, and desire to support her, well and good. But never marry her."
Sylvanus Stall, D. D.

Let the warning therefore be plain. If you value your own or your future wife's happiness, never marry a weak, sickly girl Such women have not the slightest right to marry. They become *in every case* a curse to themselves and to the man who marries them.

Marriage is first and foremost a physical union, and unless there is that stamina, that vigor in each which would indicate their ability to perform properly their part of the contract, they have not the slightest right to enter such a condition.

EXCESS DEFINED.

When this subject is broached many men will ask what is excess. How often can such indulgence be allowed and still keep within the bounds of temperance? No rule can be made for everyone. Each man must find out for himself, for what would be termed excessive in one case might be considered temperate in another.

"Many married people will give themselves up to the embrace daily, often more
than once, and that for years, But not only
its frequency, but the manner in which it is
performed, are so unnatural and studiously
licentious that the most desperate cases of
paralysis and epilepsy are frequently the direct and immediate result. Locomotor ataxia
and palsy, too, often follow in its wake."
A. T. Reinhold, Ph. D., M. D.

HEALTHY WOMAN CAN ALWAYS TELL.

"Woman is the final umpire as to its frequency.   Following her lead will usually
conduct all to matrimonial harmony ; ignor.
ing it, to discord. *Only a healthy one, however, will decide right.* A husband who tender-
ly loves a delicate wife will find no difficulty
in being continent, because he loves her too
well to subject her to what would be injurious.   Attempts have been made by legis-
lators and divines to fix definitely a limit to
the conjugal approaches which should be
binding upon all, but this is evidently im-
practicable. Generally speaking the hygienic
rule is, that after the act the person should

feel well and strong, the sleep should be sound, and the mind clear. Whenever this is not the case, when the limbs feel languid, the appetite feeble or capricious, the head ache, the intellect dull, and the faculties sluggish, then there certainly is excess, and the act should be indulged in more rarely. Those who strictly observe these rules will need no others, and will incur no danger from over-indulgence."—*Prof. O. S. Fowler.*

INSTINCT OR YOUR FEELING CAN JUDGE.

The best guide, when desirous of knowing if you indulge to excess, is your own feelings. When living under martial conditions and you seem to be lacking in energy, when your strength seems to be lessening, when that "tired feeling" becomes chronic, if you are taking precautions to follow the rules that demand regular exercise, nourishing, wholesome diet, proper bathing, and a copious supply of pure air at all times, you can at once conclude that sexual excess has something to do with your weakness.

Of course, the remedy under these circumstances is first, temperance, preferably entire abstinence in all sexual relations.

In addition to this every possible natural means for building up the physical forces, as advised further along in this book, must be regularly used.

CHAPTER V.

___

NIGHT LOSSES AND OTHER DRAINS UPON VITAL POWERS.

___

ERRONEOUS BELIEF IN REFERENCE TO THIS.

One of the most deplorable errors that the average young man has to contend with at the present time is the belief that night losses are always productive of serious ailments, that they are a sign of approaching senility, or presage insanity and other serious results. Nothing could be further from the truth. It would be difficult to find a well-sexed man who had not in one time in his life had losses of semen in this way. Under normal conditions the emission is simply a vent for the discharge of surplus semen and should in no way produce any deleterious consequences.

A PHYSICIAN'S WORDS.

"Great alarm is often expressed by patients who suffer in this way; but I am enabled to give them much relief when I mention that such emissions, occurring once in every ten or fourteen days, are in the nature of a safety valve, and are even conducive to health in persons who do not take enough exercise, and live generously. It would, however, be better for the adult to be free even from these; and I feel convinced that in one who has not allowed himself to dwell on sexual thoughts, but takes strong bodily exercise, and lives abstemiously, emissions will either not occur, or their occurrence may be looked for only very rarely. It is only when the losses or escapes take place repeatedly, attended by symptoms of prostration, with other ill consequences, that the patient should seek medical advice "—*Dr. Acton.*

Of course where the losses are of frequent occurrence they unquestionably depreciate the general vital powers, and means should be adopted to lessen their frequency. Of the means necessary for the accomplishment of this we will enter into further along in this chapter.

USUALLY CAUSED BY MASTURBATION.

These excessive nocturnal losses usually follow the habit of masturbation, and practically result from this evil. A drain is of course established if this habit is regularly indulged, and when the victim discovers its terrible consequences to mind and body and regains sufficient strength of will to renounce it, the semen that has been used to supply this drain continues to accumulate, and the amorous desire that this creates so influences the brain during sleep that lascivious dreams are produced, which usually result in this loss. Where these dreams are followed by a feeling of lassitude or extreme weariness, dizziness and general weakness, they are occurring too frequently, though it is well to remember the effect of mind over body, and that your belief in the weakening effects of these losses may be influencing your feelings in this way quite seriously. In other words, if you will at once cast aside from your mind the belief in the injurious effects of these dreams, you may not notice any of the weakening effects which seem so plain when you expect and are searching for signs of them.

ALL MEN SUFFER FROM SIMILAR LOSSES.

" But when young men are made to believe that any and all emissions are certain and

unmistakable indications of coming imbecility, the statement is both preposterous
and absurd.   Such a statement is wholly
unreliable and misleading.   After years of
acquaintance with men in all periods of life,
and after having spoken freely with many
upon the subject, the writer is frank to con-
fess that he has yet to meet the first male of
the human race, who has passed the period
of puberty and who has attained to early
manhood, who has not at some time had
such emissions, and from whom an undue
accumulation of sexual fluid has not passed
during hours of sleep in a dream of a more
or less amorous nature.

We have also carefully examined medical
authorities upon this subject, and find that
all reliable writers are agreed that such loss
of semen, if not occurring at too frequent
intervals, is not only quite general, but
seemingly natural."—*Sylvanus Stall, D.D.*

MEDICAL FAKIRS AND THEIR PREY.

This idea that these losses are always injurious, and that they never occur under any
circumstances when enjoying prefectly nor-

mal state, has been spread broadcast by the patent-medicine fakirs, who live by robbing the public just as leeches feast on the vitality of other animals.

Think of the vast sums annually spent for their various remedies, which are supposed to bring to the wasted victims of these complaints that strength and virility which have been frittered away. The amount would almost pay the national debt. And do these remedies cure? Do they ever benefit? The manufacturers of these base impositions no doubt profit by them, but no one else. If the evil ended with the fleecing of the unwary, the consequence would not be serious, but thousands are buoyed with false hope after reading of the wonderful cures advertised by these frauds, whose proper home is in a penitentiary.

BLIND SEARCH FOR A CURE.

Because of the belief that these spurious remedies are the only available method of cure, the victims have no opportunity to become interested in natural means which would bring health and strength in every instance where such a result was possible; and naturally they go on, year after year, trying one quack remedy after another, until the grave opens and ends their miseries.

MURDERS COMMITTED.

No cry of murder goes up at the poor victim's funeral. He is laid peacefully away with loud lamentations and regrets at the intervention of Divine Providence. But who is to blame for this murder—this poisoning by slow degrees of a life that might have been useful and prolonged? Enumerate all the deaths that occur in a usual serious war through diseases and other causes and multiply it by one hundred, and it would probably closely approximate the actual number who annually lose their lives through the causes mentioned above. We have every precaution to protect the weak and the ignorant from robbery or assault, but who on this earth are protecting the fragile, inexperienced, nervous wrecks from being robbed, physically and financially, by the quacks and should-be convicts, who hire the space and reputation of the most renowed newspapers and periodicals to assist them in their nefarious business?

NEWSPAPERS SUPPLY THEIR COLUMNS TO THIEVES

In one part of a prominent newspaper a most terrible arraignment of some trust or public enemy will appear, but in the same paper, under the head of advertisements, one can read the most seductive and insinuating offers to those suffering from "hidden weaknesses," etc., etc. The editors and managers no doubt wonder how enough victims can be caught to pay for such large advertising bills, but somehow they seem to forget that these same victims are as capable of suffering as those who are injured by the trusts. It is the appalling ignorance of the masses on these subjects with which every adult should be familiar, that enables the blood-suckers to ply their trade. Do not under any circumstances allow the fakirs to get you in their clutches.

RULES FOR LESSENING NIGHT LOSSES.

If you feel that night losses are becoming too frequent, adopt the following special rules and give particular attention to the other rules found in this work, and you can depend upon a complete recovery, though remember that it will take time to accomplish this. As to just how often emissions must occur in order to be considered too frequent, it is exceedingly difficult to determine. The sexual power of man varies most widely in different individuals, and what would be considered excess in one might be extreme temperance in another The best guide is to be sure that the symptons of weakness which follows this loss are not in the mind, but are an actual physical reality. When sure of this you can nearly always depend on the conclusion that the loss is becoming excessive.

WHEN LOSSES ARE EXCESSIVE.

Some writers claim that a loss once each week is excessive; others that twice each week in some men would not be considered so.

Judge for yourself in your own particulaı case, though if the rules here given are accurately followed, if there is an excessive loss, it will soon begin to decrease.

Be careful never to cover yourself too heavily during sleep. Better wake up cold at times than to induce undue warmth.

Never sleep on your back. If you are in the habit of doing this, wear a belt with some small article attached against your back so that the moment you turn over on your back during sleep you will be awakened.

CULTIVATE A LOVE FOR COLD WATER.

Do not under any circumstances neglect the practice of gradually inuring yourself to the use of cold water morning and evening, though a complete sitz bath will be found of especial advantage after exercise on rising.

Take up regular exercise, though be very moderate at first.

If the exercise is overdone it will tend to aggravate your trouble. Deep breathing and long walks can especially be commended.

Don't over-eat.

It is a hundred times preferable to eat too little than to eat too much. Eat nourishing, appetizing foods only. Eat slowly, masticate thoroughly.

Keep the bowels regular by using laxative

foods. If this does not suffice, read chapter on Constipation and follow suggestions given there.

Don't worry. (Read chapter on Mental Influence.)

Don't crowd your brain with lewd thoughts. The more you allow your thoughts to dwell on these subjects, the more semen is accumulated, and the more your trouble will be aggravated. Keep the mind busy with some active and interesting occupation.

KEEP THE MIND CLEAN.

"When the mind is permitted to dwell unduly upon sexual subjects, the secretions become more rapid than is designed, the system is drained, and more injury is done by the impure thought that produces this result than by the dream which attends the emptying of the sacs which are flooded with this vital fluid more rapidly than it can be re-absorbed for use throughout the entire system. Thus it will be seen that the purity of the mind is both of primary and vital importance."—*Sylvanus Stall, D. D.*

CHAPTER VI.

PROMISCUOUS INTERCOURSE.

USUALLY NOTHING BUT LUST.

No reasoning man who carefully investigates the subject can avoid condemning promiscuous intercourse. In many cases it is almost as unnatural as masturbation. The woman who allows promiscuous privileges in this way cares nothing for a man. There is absolutely no natural reciprocation on the part of the female. His feeling for her is nothing more than the lowest, the most bestial passion. It is simply *lust, lust, lust*, of the lowest order. The female endures the embrace for whatever she may gain. Such relations are unnatural and therefore productive of both physical and mental deterioration. This would be the unquestionable result even if no disease is acquired, and think of the terrible risk incurred in this way!

"Promiscuous intercourse leads to gonorrhœa, gleet, syphilis, stricture, diseased offspring, childlessness, and many other evils. Almost the entire civilized race is to-day tainted with venereal poison. If we imagine vitality divided into equal portions, each item may be looked upon as canceled by an act of cohabitation. Then it is obvious that the more frequent these acts of intercourse, the sooner the stock of vital power must be exhausted."—*A. F. Reinhold, Ph. D., M. D.*

TERRIBLE PENALTIES FOR THIS SIN.

Nature has set a price upon fornication that none can afford to give. She takes her pay in physical power, in health. It is against her laws, and those who break the laws must pay the price.

No man who makes a habit of visiting this class of women ever escapes for long, and some of the diseases are of the most loathsome character. Go to any of the hospitals and see the myriads of sufferers from these ailments that actually at times eat the flesh from the bones, leaving great open sores that are healed only by death.

CAUSES LOATHSOME VENEREAL DISEASES.

"God in nature condemns sexual depravities as the most utterly abominable in His holy sight of all others, and affixes to them the seal of His uttermost reprobation, by appending to them pains and penalties more painful, and loathsomeness more disgusting than to any other sins and vices. Natural expression always tells the truth, and nothing but the truth, though by no means the whole truth here, for that is impossible, even by this Heaven's most eloquent orator. A strong man or woman slowly atoning, by lingering, agonizing moments, hours, days and months, till a protracted death finally closes upon the scene, the author never has seen, never desires to see. Other pens, more vivid, have attempted this painful description, only confessedly to fall far short of its awful realities. What feverish days! What restless nights! What agonizing aches and pains in every bone, and muscle, and nerve! What eyes rolling and glaring and protruding, as if internal agonies were pushing them out of their sockets! An awful stench nauseates beyond any power of description. A putrid human carcass—beast does not, cannot suffer this—is livid with poison! Running sores here, there, everywhere,

ejecting excretions how utterly disgusting!"
—*Prof. O. S. Fowler.*

FINE ATHLETES BECOME WRECKS.

The writer has seen many a strong, fine athletic man brought down to a physical wreck by these terrible diseases. Even gonorrhea, which is usually apparently cured in a short time, often brings on complications and results in serious loss of physical and sexual power.

FEARFUL WARNING FOR ALL.

"If men whose abnormal desires lead them into the ways of promiscuous intercourse could but see some one or more of the vic tims to be found at all times in any of the large hospitals—the foul, loathsome ulcer; the poison eating away gradually, slowly, but surely, the flesh; the eyes gone, the nose destroyed, giving the face a most hideous aspect; the bones of the skull eaten, exposing the brain; the mark of manhood obliterated altogether, a loathsome, living death—they would think twice before venturing into the meshes of her whose 'feet take hold on hell.'

The breaking of no other human law entails on the wrong-doer such fearfully prompt, repulsive and incurable penalties as does the unnatural one of miscellaneous intercourse. The very first transgression ofttimes devel ops the poison of syphilis, the non-desire for which may be inferred from what one of the most distinguished of French surgeons has said: 'I would not have a chancre of the size of a pin's head on my person for all Paris.'"
—*John Cowan, M. D.*

DESTRUCTIVE EFFECTS OF USUAL TREATMENT

Any of these sexual diseases unquestion-ably causes a serious loss of sexual strength, not only on account of the general physical decline that accompanies and follows them, but the ordinary treatment used is often ex-tremely harsh (usually far more so than it should be) and the strong drugs, ejections, etc., that are used to effect a cure, leave traces of their weakening influences often years after their use has been discontinued.

Regardless of what opinion may be formed as to desirabilty of absolute continence, no reasoning process can possibly cause a man to conclude that promiscuous intercourse is either beneficial or desirable. This conclusion cannot be avoided, even if one is laboring under the delusion that he is too careful to acquire any of the terrible diseases that are the main penalties for the infraction of these laws.

CHAPTER VII.

TOBACCO—ITS DESTRUCTIVE EFFECT ON SEXUAL POWERS.

SOMETIMES DIRECT CAUSE OF IMPOTENCE.

There is a uniformity of opinion among all writers on this subject as to the effects of tobacco on sexual powers. The writer has heard of numerous cases where it has actually been the direct cause of impotence. One particular case is remembered where a patient was being treated for entire loss of power in this way. The physician had prescribed the usual remedies, and had been treating the patient for some time without any sign of improvement. One day while reading a work on the evil results of smoking, he was quite surprised to note the special injury which the author of the work claimed that smoking produced on the sexual powers. He, of course, naturally realized that the influence of smoking was far from desirable, but did not consider it as injurious as the author claimed. He remembered that the patient whom he was then treating was a great smoker, and that he had told him on one or two occasions that his improvement might be more rapid if he would be more moderate in this habit.

ACTUAL EXPERIMENTS PROVED ITS EFFECTS.

The author's theories appealed to him and he determined to enjoin entire abstinence from smoking upon his patient and to watch the result. In less than a month the patient's long-lost powers returned and the physician allowed him to resume his cigars. The result was that in a short time his old trouble appeared, and ultimately he found that cigars must be avoided or else a chronic condition of impotence would continue.

INFLUENCE ON THE NERVES.

The use of tobacco, either smoking or chewing, has an enormous influence on the nervous system. Nothing proves this so emphatically as the intense, almost overpowering, craving which is induced after the use of the weed becomes a habit. It benumbs and destroys the finer delicacy of the nerves. Any influence on the general nervous system of course affects the organs of sex directly, for, as explained before, they are a part of the nervous system.

DECREASES STRENGTH AND SENSITIVENESS OF EVERY POWER.

"To one who has not attained his entire growth, the use of tobacco stunts the body and dwarfs the muscles, making them flabby and weak. When used in excess, tobacco greatly affects the vision. Physicians who make the treatment of the eye a specialty tell us that when they use the magnifying lens, and throw the light in upon the retina of the eye, they can tell immediately when one is addicted to the excessive use of tobacco. It also deadens the hearing, greatly affects the heart, producing palpitation, and when used regularly, in large quantities, results in producing what is called "tobacco heart." The results of either smoking or chewing can often be noticed in its effects upon the nerves, rendering the individual both nervous and irritable, even to small provocation. Surgeons tell us that their experience in the operating room has developed the fact that men who are addicted to the use of tobacco quite generally suffer a lack of manly fortitude, and are noticeably cowardly under the severe trial of a surgical operation. Tobacco discolors the teeth, makes the breath offensive, excites the glands which secrete the saliva, and tends to produce dyspepsia, low spirits, a pale face, and an emaciated form. It also tends to produce dizziness, rush of blood to the head, palpitation of the heart, loss of memory, and a diseased condition of the mouth. Such results have been noted in the death of prominent persons, such as General Grant' and many others."—*Sylvanus Stall, D. D.*

DESTROYS FINER DELICACY OF THE NERVES.

Smoking, or the use of tobacco in any form, therefore, must be avoided if the highest degree of strength and delicacy of the nerves are desired. This nervous vigor carries with it all the intensity and strength of superb sexual power, and any deteriorating influence will similarly affect this power.

It is also a well-known fact that smoking has a weakening influence upon the entire physical organism. Numerous instances have occurred where it was proven to be the direct cause of serious digestive troubles. But the most stubborn argument against the use of tobacco is the fact that all athletes in training entirely avoid it. No matter how much they have been addicted to the habit, always when the time arrives for them to begin the work which is to build the highest degree of health and strength, smoking is immediately and absolutely tabooed. Its effect on endurance is most marked, as a smoker, just as a hard drinker, after one or two strenuous efforts is usually entirely exhausted.

HOW TO BREAK THE HABIT.

It is an easy matter to break the habit if the same method is adopted as advised for curing the liquor habit—that is, gradually to lessen the use day by day. (See chapter on Alcohol and Other Stimulants—Their Destructive Effects.)

The practice, too, of following accurately

in detail the instructions for building up the nervous and muscular powers is of just as much importance in ridding one of this habit as in the cure of the alcohol habit, and if you desire to be young again, if you desire to experience the joys, elasticity and intensity that accompany the powers and exuberance of extreme virility, the use of tobacco must positively be avoided.

CHAPTER VIII.

THE DESTRUCTIVE EFFECTS OF ALCOHOL AND OTHER STIMULANTS

HEALTH AND SEXUAL VIGOR CO-EXISTENT.

"Along with sexual health and calmness go good general health and general quietness of the nerves. Nothing is so detrimental to this condition as the use of stimulants and narcotics."—*Prof. O. S. Fowler.*

Next to sexual excess or kindred unnatural drains the greatest cause of impotence is unquestionably the use of alcohol and other stimulants, which act like a spur on every organ of the body.

No true strength can ever be produced by any stimulant. It is always false strength, and is created at the expense of vital power, and really assists just that much in lessening the true strength of all parts of the body.

ALCOHOL LESSENS SEXUAL POWER.

"It is scarcely necessary that we should say anything about the injurious effects of liquors of all kinds upon the reproductive organs. It is well known that drunkards and tipplers are easily robbed of sexual power. The ancient proverb says, 'Venus is drowned in Bacchus.' Shakespeare aptly displays his marvelous range of information in the play 'Macbeth,' where the porter says to Macduff, 'Drinking provokes the desire, but it takes away the performance: it makes him, and it mars him; it sets him on, and it takes him off; it persuades him, and it disheartens him,' etc. Manliness and virile power in their best development are impossible to those who use liquor of any kind in any quantity."—*Sylvanus Stall, D. D.*

Physical vigor and sexual vigor are companions. You will nearly always find them together in the same person. Anything that tends to build up one will increase the other in power. Therefore take a lesson from prize-fighters and all other athletes in training for a contest, which means training to reach the highest degree of health, and leave all stimulants absolutely alone.

EASY METHOD FOR BREAKING THE HABIT.

Of course, if you are in the habit of taking a certain amount of alcoholic liquors each day, the writer does not ask that you immediately cease this indulgence, though if one is possessed of the necessary will-power to do this recovery will be much quicker because of the abstinence.

This method, however, requires great strength of will, and is not by any means necessary. You can be cured without suffering from this wild craving.

The writer will tell you just how it can be done.

First take up the method of treatment advised here. Read *very, very* carefully the chapter on Diet; follow accurately the instructions as to exercise, bathing, clothing, fresh air, etc., etc.

After you have begun to follow these rules gradually lessen by one every day or two the number of daily drinks. When you are taking only one each day, try to make it one every other day, then one every third day, after which you will probably find no difficulty in leaving it alone altogether. The desire for a stimulant of any kind always indicates a lowered condition of the general health, and under the influence of natural means for building up the physical forces but little difficulty will be found in breaking the stimulant habit if the required efforts are made. The great importance of using infinite care never to over-eat, and not to eat at any time unless very hungry, cannot be too strongly emphasized in this trouble.

OVER-EATING PRODUCES CRAVINGS FOR A STIMULANT.

One of the greatest causes of the craving for a stimulant is over-eating, and this fact must be clearly understood if you are desirous of ridding yourself of this slavery. Of course, the moderate use of alcohol can be continued and a certain amount of benefit will be secured by following the exercises and other advice found here, but if you desire all the intensity and power of the emotional and sexual nature that you will no doubt remember to have possessed when in fullness of early youth the stimulant habit must be absolutely avoided. You cannot acquire all the marvelous delicacy and intensity of this superb power unless its benumbing influence is totally withdrawn.

"The use of liquor destroys health, disfigures the body, ruins the nervous system, dethrones the reason, produces insanity, becomes the parent of idiocy; it blunts the finer feelings and sensibilities; it fills our poor-houses with paupers and crowds our prisons with criminals; it breaks the hearts of parents and pauperizes helpless women and innocent children; it leads to vice and violence, and plunges its victims into temporal and eternal ruin."—*Sylvanus Stall, D.D.*

Chapter IX.

ELECTRIC–BELT FAKE.

ABSOLUTELY NO MERIT IN THIS MEANS.

Unquestionably the use of patent medicines is gradually declining. The public has been deceived and robbed of money and health so much by these rank fakes that it is beginning gradually to lose faith in the ridiculous claims of cures made by the proprietors of these so-called remedies. But with the decline of the use of this means of cure there has arisen a "do-nothing" cure, which, in the form of electric belts, though not as bad as many harmful drugs, is still dangerous, for the reason that it lulls the sufferer into false security, by impressing him with the idea that he is "doing something" for his ailment. These electric belt fakirs are up to date. Nearly every one of their conspicuous advertisements contain large, artistically drawn figures of athletic men in a physical condition that no electric belt could assist, even in the slightest degree, to bring about.

RIDICULOUS CLAIMS OF CURES.

The various owners of these fake cures usually make the same ridiculous claims for their belts as are made by patent-medicine venders, namely, that the mere use of their appliance will effect a cure, that the disease, which in every case is brought about by the violation of the great health laws, can be remedied by merely applying their belts. According to their claims, there is no need to give the slightest attention to the cause of the trouble, since the belts will in every case produce the desired results; though some of the more intelligent give advice, the following of which often effects a cure, that of course, is credited to the electric belt.

MAY CURE IMAGINARY DISEASES.

Electric belts never have cured and never will cure disease of any kind. They may cure many diseases that have existed in the imagination only, or they may produce benefit by creating a more hopeful mental state, but a condition of actual disease can no more be cured by an electric belt than the body can be kept clean without water.

Of course, these belts are mostly recommended for weakness of the organs of sex, and indeed in some cases they may stimulate these organs. If this result is produced, impotence is produced just that much quicker, because of this unnatural stimulation. There is but one proper means of building strength in this way, and that is to strengthen the entire muscular and nervous system by regular exercise.

WORK FOR RESULTS DESIRED.

Stop trying to get something for nothing. Leave electric belts alone, unless you are anxious to rid yourself of money. If you want health, strength, the virility, vitality of complete, fully developed manhood or womanhood, work for this superb condition. You can secure it in no other way.

CHAPTER X.

THE INFLUENCE OF ABSOLUTE CONTINENCE.

MEN ARE NOT UNIFORM.

Man's physical, mental and moral self, partly inherited, but principally developed by the environments of early life, guides his actions and creates the conditions under which he must live in order to attain the highest degree of physical and mental perfection. No two individuals are exactly alike. That which means happiness to one might mean most abject misery to another. In every species of the animal world outside of the human animal there exists a certain degree of uniformity in physique and mentality; but the physical and mental traits and powers of men vary as widely as do the quickness, suppleness and mental acuteness of the tiger when compared to the clumsiness, apparent stupidity, and phlegmatic temperament of the hippopotamus. With this fact clear, would any intelligent person dare to lay down rules for all to follow indiscriminately?

CHASTITY—IS IT HARMFUL?

This is a much-mooted question! The average physician will tell you that a man is better and stronger if temperate indulgences of a proper character are afforded, but most of the writers along sexual lines strenuously defend one's ability to remain absolutely continent all through life without suffering the slightest from this abstinence.

It is undoubtedly considered desirable to remain continent until the fullness of complete maturity has been reached, and the more deficiency there is in those powers necessary to a perfect man or woman, the less harm there will result from a life of absolute continence. Some, no doubt, could be continent all their life and still apparently enjoy the average powers, but their ability thus to deviate from Nature's laws with comparative impunity indicates that the completeness of fully developed manhood has never been reached—that the powers which accompany perfect maturity are still dormant.

MANHOOD NEVER REACHED.

Some men—usually for the lack of physical training—never grow to complete manhood. They practically remain children all their lives—children in mind and in body: weak and wavering in their desires and in their mental and physical individuality. Can we say that one's brain is mature merely because it has existed a certain number of years? Is it not rather the training which the brain receives that speeds it on to maturity? It is the same with the body, which must be trained, strengthened, developed, or it will remain childish in its immaturity, and will lack to an extreme degree that hardy vigor which could easily have been acquired through proper physical culture.

PREMATURELY DEVELOPED SEXUAL POWERS.

Unquestionably, where a boy grows into manhood without the contaminating thoughts and deteriorating physical and mental influences that result from masturbation, he can go through life and remain continent without suffering any particularly noticeable inconvenience, and if *mentally satisfied with his condition*, can probably enjoy nearly the same energy and success that might have been his under more normal conditions. We must remember, however, the enormous influence of mind over body. A man's ability to remain permanently continent depends largely on his mental condition. We must admit that the average human being of the present day is born under conditions that tend to aggravate or develop to an abnormal extent the sexual instinct. But few marriages are based on right lines. Excess is the rule in nearly every case, and this sexual excess is usually continued even at the time the child is forming and growing into life. When this is considered, can one wonder at the premature development of the sexual instinct in children? And then comes the prudish silence along sexual lines, which is so significant to a growing, thinking boy. It arouses his curiosity, his interest. This, combined with the stimulating diet adopted in most civilized homes, soon results in calling a boy's most serious attention to this sexual part of his nature, and this instinct is consequently developed prematurely, causing him to learn and practice self-abuse often long before puberty has been passed.

CONTINENCE RARE IN THOSE WHO ONCE FALL.

The writer has seen and heard of instances of absolute continence being maintained by men who have somehow escaped the conditions that lead up to self-abuse, but he has never yet known a man to lead a permanently continent life after once contracting this habit. It seems that, after a drain of this kind upon the system has once been established, the sexual passions develop prematurely, and often become too strong to be ignored far earlier in life than they would if normal conditions had existed. Therefore much of the sexual intemperance met with at the present is really due originally to the habit of masturbation, which, in nine cases out of ten, is made possible by the worse than criminal neglect of parents.

MARRIAGE A NECESSITY.

Every law of nature emphasizes the necessity for marriage; animal life everywhere gives evidence to this. The highest degree of attainable physical perfection can certainly never be acquired unless this condition is entered at the proper period of life. It may be put off; the day of its consummation may be delayed; but it must come before the powers of manhood and womanhood are on the wane, or one will never be able to taste its joys and its benefits in the brightness and strength of full maturity. Successful men nearly always marry; many of them are fathers of large families. The founding of a home with one for whom there exists a reverential love, is usually one of the first steps to fame and fortune. It makes one feel settled in life; it confines the efforts towards a more definite goal. The seriousness and responsibilities of home life give strength to the will and steadiness to life's aims and to the powers of persistence.

MENTAL INFLUENCE.

The environments of life, mental, moral and physical, influence to a remarkable degree that element in the human mind and body which indicates the age or time when marriage should be consummated. If deeply absorbed in a profession, or in study of any kind, with no time or desire to allow the mind to dwell on anything of a sentimental nature, the development of sex is retarded, and should this complete absorption long continue, this dormant condition may remain all through life, though this is a rare occurrence. Many become so engrossed in life's duties or ambitions that love goes by them year after year, until some face, some sympathetic individuality, appeals to them, and awakens to life their desire for the tenderness and companionship of the marital relation.

WHEN TO MARRY.

Now the reader may ask, at what age should I marry? First, when you have attained complete maturity; second, after you have met one for whom you have a deep, reverential love, which, of course, must be returned with the same fervor and strength. But suppose I meet no one for whom I have this reverential love? you may ask. Well, do not marry until you do experience this. Marriage is sanctified, not by the ceremony which binds the pair in a civil contract, but by love; it is made holy, reverential, by the

intensity and thorough unselfishness of this
love. When this exalted affection exists,
and is not degraded and destroyed by being
animalized, one can be carried on the wave
of this great happiness far beyond his ordinary capacities, can be made capable of that
which, under ordinary circumstances, would
not only be improbable, but impossible.
Marriage under these proper conditions
èlevates, ennobles, strengthens, increases the
self-confidence, and no man, no woman, can
be developed to all the fullness of attainable power unless he or she enters this
natural condition.

SEXUAL APPETITE CANNOT BE IGNORED.

No one can question the conclusion that
the sexual appetite was made to be satisfied,
and there comes a time in the life of every
man when in order to go onward and upward
to the attainment of his highest powers, of
his greatest strength, mental and physical,
he must be under this perfectly natural
influence. The age, of course, when this
occurs differs quite widely, being governed
largely by one's mental and physical condi-

tion and previous environments. It would arrive sooner in a man who had awakened his sexual nature to life by abnormal habits, or in a man who had come in contact with one of the opposite sex who had strongly aroused a desire for the marital relation. The sexual appetite is entirely under mental control. It will sleep on for years if the brain would not call it into life. No reasoner along these lines can claim that a normal man, in possession of a strongly sexed nature, can be absolutely continent during his entire life and still acquire all the energy of body and power of mind and intensity of emotions that might have been his had he provided proper legitimate means of following the natural desire of his sexual instinct.

"MAN WAS NOT MADE TO LIVE ALONE."

This Biblical maxim is unquestionably true in nearly every case, and when its truth is disregarded in the life of a normal man, he fails to reach his highest degree of attainable physical and mental excellence.

A prominent writer along sexual lines, who strenuously maintains that extreme continence carries with it no evil effects, states that "the purest, noblest and most unselfish aspirations and purposes derive their strength and being from the sweet influences which have their beginning and their continuance in this power which draws men and women in happy and holy wedlock.

"Where life has been untarnished by the social evil, the sexual impulse marches like a mighty conqueror, arousing and marshaling the mightiest human powers in every department of man's nature. It formulates his purpose, quickens his imagination, and calls into exercise his united powers in the attainment of the world's greatest and grandest achievements in art, in letters, in inventions, in philosophy. It strengthens every faculty, quickens every power."

SUPERB MANHOOD WILL NOT ALLOW
CONTINUED CONTINENCE.

If you are not a man; if though fully grown, you are still a child and always expect to remain one; you can be continent all through life without suffering to any appreciable extent. But if you are a man in every sense, possessing the complete powers of body and mind which accompany this state of maturity, with all the faculties fully alive, with all the emotions tingling with the intensity of their strength, with the glory and ripeness of life, of health and of strength stirring your senses, the strength of your desire for the marital relation will be too strong to resist, and Nature has willed that this should be so.

CHAPTER XI.

WHY MARRIAGE SOMETIMES WRECKS.

ALL INTERESTED IN MARRIAGE.

The attention given marital troubles at the present time indicates beyond question that it is a subject of paramount interest and importance. It appeals to every one. " It strikes home," for, although all are not married, there are few who do not look forward to this condition—or backward at it. The various theories that are advanced as to the cause of marital unhappiness by philosophers throughout the world would fill thousands of volumes. But the writer has often wondered how many of these theories expressed the real opinions of the writers. He cannot believe that they fail to see the real cause of marital unhappiness, or that it is their desire to deceive, but to his mind it is plain that divorces, and by far the larger majority of the unhappy marriages, are made possible by abnormal physical conditions and excesses, resulting largely from gross ignorance of those laws with which every adult human being should be familiar.

MARRIAGE A PHYSICAL UNION.

Marriage was a well-known and popular institution long before the human race ever thought of refinement, of civilization and its varying environments. The brute husband was able to hold his human property by a power stronger than all earthly forces; that is, mere physical attraction. Marriage was then entirely a physical union. It was contracted and continued on that basis. There was but little ceremony about it—usually none. A man desired a woman, and if this desire was mutual, he took her. Sometimes even her acceptance was not required This was marriage at that time. Though we have advanced intellectually—though man has made tremendous strides in all that pertains to the graces of culture and refinement, a true marriage still must have physical attraction for its foundation, and is primarily and fundamentally a physical union.

PARENTAL LOVE A PHYSICAL INSTINCT.

Of course, all must admit that there is supposed to be something higher in modern marriages than mere physical love. There is at times a love so intense, so exalted, that it is akin to the worship a religious enthusiast is supposed to extend to God ; but all this great love is made possible by the previous existence of intense physical love. If marriage could be based on reverential respect, or any other regard that has no physical aspect, man and man, or woman and woman, could marry with the same felicity and propriety that the sexes are now mated. But the mere thought of uniting marriage with such conditions is repugnant—and rightly so. But is it necessarily a disgrace for marriage to be founded on physical attraction ? One of the most admirable traits in the human character is the love of a mother for her child, and the reader may be shocked when we say that such regard is mere animal or physical love; for the grandest exhibition of the sacrificial spirit of parental love can be found among the lower animals. An animal that is as timid as a hare, under ordinary circumstances, will often fight with the frenzy of a man-eating tiger when its young are to be protected. Therefore, why belittle animal love? In its noblest form it is one of the grandest of all human passions or human instincts.

PHYSICAL CONDITION OF THOSE ENTERING MATRIMONY.

Admitting that marriage is fundamentally a physical institution, that whatever the exalted height of the regard existing between the contracting parties, it is made possible first by physical attraction, then call to mind the average physical condition of those who have entered, and are still entering, the holy bonds of matrimony. When such facts are viewed, the great wonder is not why there are so few, but why there are so many happy marriages under such abnormal conditions. Although the men are far from the physical standard that they should approximate, the principal fault is to be found in the female sex, for as far as the marital relations are concerned, it is the woman who should have control, and should be blessed with that physical excellence, which will supply the finer instincts essential under such circumstances.

GREAT PHYSICAL DEFICIENCY OF WOMAN.

The female human animal should be as strong in proportion to the male as is the female of lower animals. That the average woman falls far below this standard, no one will deny. The female cat, dog, horse or lion is but little weaker than the male of their own species, and in a race can usually run about as fast as the male. Woman should be as strong in comparison with man.

" Our young women, how miserably sexed, physically. Few are two-thirds grown. Most are dwarfed, rendered too small to be of much practical account, by excessive brain and deficient bodily action. Scan the forms of these pocket Venuses. Nearly all are deficient in bust and pelvis, meagre in face and limb, narrow and round-shouldered, humpbacked, crooked-backed, stooping, too fat, unless too lean, with their breast bones caved in, short ribs meeting or overlapping, bowels small or knotted; faces painted, besides. What a damaging confession that they need

to paint? Yet how awfully they look without, and even with? And use cologne in
addition, thus telling all within smelling
distance that they lack that balmy perfume
which is coincident with sexuality. ONE-
FOURTH HAVE CROOKED SPINES."—
Prof. O. S. Fowler.

PHYSICAL WEAKNESS CAUSE OF MARITAL MISERIES.

The lack of physical excellence, more
especially among women, is unquestionably
one of the greatest causes of marital unhappiness. Although men are supposed to
select their wives, *woman in reality does the
selecting,* and if all her physical forces are not
developed to their full completeness, she has
not the acuteness of discrimination in sexual
selection that she would possess under more
normal conditions. Hence she often selects
a man for a husband, not because she loves
him with all the devotion, intensity and
power that should accompany every true
marriage, but because he will enable her to
advance socially, or to satisfy other ambitions. In an insipid way, she may believe

that she loves some other man more than the one she marries, but in her eyes he may not be her equal, or may not be able to give her the position and influence desired, and as the strength, emotions and power of a true woman are still dormant in her undeveloped body, she is incapable of loving any one to any great degree of intensity, and therefore does not allow love to influence her choice. What pitiable objects such women are? They go through life cold, heartless, pitiless, unfeeling creatures. That divine desire of every true woman's soul for motherhood, for the prattling voices of their own lovely children, they never experience. They are not women —not men. The world is made darker, gloomier, and more severe because of their influence at times, but rarely, if ever, is it made better.

FINELY SEXED WOMEN MARRY FOR LOVE ONLY.

Marriage for position or money, or to satisfy other desires than love, is made possible simply and entirely by the lack of that virile power which accompanies superb physical health.   A finely sexed, fully-developed, womanly woman could no more marry without love than fire could mingle with water. Her whole physical, mental and moral being would cry out with repugnance and loathing against such a union.

WOMEN LACK PROTECTING INSTINCT OF SEX.

As a first step in marital unhappiness, because of the lack of physical excellence, many women contract loveless marriages, which always start and end unhappily. For the need of this same physical power, which carries with it the normal instinct necessary to protect a woman from the more gross passions of her marital partner, the life of many a married couple becomes a most harrassing existence, and in addition the woman suffers most serious physical tortures from the effects of unnatural excesses. There is nothing that predisposes a woman so strongly towards that which is right, natural and moral as the finer instincts of superb animal power. Such a woman is moral because her every desire, her every instinct is in favor of morality. Such a woman has no difficulty in finding and—what is more important—keeping a husband, for the simple reason that she respects the strong instincts of her nature, and forces her husband to do likewise, thus retaining and increasing day by day his respect and his love.

WEAK WOMEN UNFIT FOR MARITAL RELATIONS.

"Those women who are pale and nervous, who are without a natural appetite, unable to do any active work, or enjoy any vigorous recreation without being constantly out of breath, who are faint and weak, always complaining of pain in their back, and many other symptoms which are inseparably connected with female weakness, are not partially, but totally, unfitted for the marriage relation, and the man who marries such a woman not only makes her miserable, but himself also, and after a few years awakens to the fact that he has made the greatest mistake of his life."—*Sylvanus Stall, D.D.*

NATURE'S LAWS OUTRAGED IN MARRIAGE.

The entire conventional idea of marriage and the duties of a wife to her husband are

abnormal, and unquestionably these perverted theories have done much towards
bringing about the unsatisfactory matrimonial condition now almost universal. The
civil ceremony is supposed to give a man
every privilege he may desire. The wife is
supposed to be subjected to his every wish.
The laws of Nature, or the laws of God, war-
rants no such conclusion. In fact, it is plain
that the wishes of the wife should be paramount—that the husband should be subjected
to and controlled by her. When this outrage
to women and the plain laws of nature, in
her total subjection to man in marital life, is
fully realized, one of the principal causes of
diseases peculiar to her sex is plain to any
unprejudiced reasoner.

FALSE CONCLUSIONS IN MARRIAGE.

How many thousands of young women,
apparently in good health, enter the realms
of matrimony, and as a result find that their
health of body and mind has been sacrificed.
This should not be. It is usually caused by
an undeveloped sexual instinct, and by the
perverted impression that marriage means

total subjection to the wishes of another. On the "rocks" of this false conclusion are shattered the happiness, health and future prospects of thousands of married couples. Herein lies the paramount importance of superb physical health. Notwithstanding the influence that may be imposed on a woman by what she may have cause to believe is her duty, she will not stoop to anything that will outrage her physical instinct if she possesses all the power, beauty and health conjoined to superb, wholesome womanhood.

MEN SHOULD BEWARE OF CORSET WRECKS.

That diaphragm-breathing and tight lacing are most ruinous to women and their offspring is self-evident. No evil equals that of curtailing this maternal supply of breath; nor does anything do this as effectually as tight lacing. If it were merely a female folly, or if its ravages were confined to its perpetrators, it might be passed unrebuked; but it strikes a deadly blow at the very life of the race. By girting in the lungs, stomach and diaphragm, it cripples every one of the life-manufacturing functions, impairs circulation, impedes muscular action, and lays siege to the child-bearing citadel itself. It often destroys germinal life before birth, or soon after, by most effectually cramping, inflaming, and weakening the vital apparatus, and stopping the flow of life at its fountain head. It takes the lives of tens of thousands before they marry, and so effectually weakens and diseases as ultimately to cause the death of millions more.

TIGHT LACING DESTROYS WOMANHOOD.

"No tongue can tell, no finite mind conceive, he misery it has occasioned, nor the number of deaths, directly and indirectly, of young women, bearing mothers, and weakly infants it has occasioned; besides those millions on millions it has caused to drag out a short but wretched existence. If this murderous practice continues another generation, it will bury all the middle and upper class of women and children, and leave propogation to the coarse-grained but healthy lower. Most alarmingly has it already deteriorated our very race in physical strength, power of constitution, energy, and talents. Reader, how many of your weaknesses, pains, headaches, nervous affections, internal difficulties, and wretched feelings, are caused by your own or mother's corset-strings? Such mother's deserve execration.

"Let men who had rather bury than raise their children, marry tight-lacers; but those who would rear a healthy, talented, happy family, to bless their mature life, nurse their declining years, and perpetuate their name and race among men, should choose those naturally full-chested; for such will be likely to live long, and bear vigorous children. Those who would not have their souls rent asunder by the premature death of wife and children, are solemnly warned not to marry small waists; for such must of necessity die young, and bear few and feeble offsprings. You women who are willing to exchange the rosy cheek of health for laced pallor, the full round form of natural beauty for the poor, scrawny, sunken, haggard, almost ghastly figure of those who lace, or break the heart of husband and friends by your premature death, after agonizing yourselves by thus causing your children's death, till you exclaim in nervous agony, 'Oh, wretched life that I live,' besides dying before your time, lace on tighter and tighter, and keep laced up night and day, till your life wheels cease to move.

"Bachelors, make 'natural waists or no wives' your motto, and frown down this fashion your patronage fosters. Women will cease to lace when you show preference to good-sized waists. Let all condemn this race ruining custom."—*Prof. O. S. Fowler.*

MARRY A WOMAN—NOT A CORSETED SEXLESS NONENTITY.

The paramount importance of selecting a woman for a wife who possesses in the highest degree that physical vigor which denotes strong sexual instinct cannot be too strongly emphasized. It is well known that but few marriages are happy, but if one were able to view the inside conditions of those who do enjoy marital bliss, the facts would indicate that the woman possesses a strong sexual instinct, and that she compelled her husband to respect this instinct, thus debilitating excesses were avoided.

Catharine Beecher says in her book on Female Ailments, as to the proportion of women diseased sexually within her extensive observation and careful personal inquiry, that it exceeds twenty-nine in every thirty. My own average is, that not one woman in one hundred has a fair amount of sexual vigor, and that at least nine in every ten, if not nineteen in, every twenty, are more or less prostrated, or else actually diseased sexually.

SEXUAL INSTINCT NECESSARY TO MARITAL HAPPINESS.

To a strongly sexed woman there are periods when intercourse should be repugnant, and if her instinct does not indicate these periods, and if she does not respect them and compel her husband to do likewise, there is small chance for happiness in such a marriage. Marriage under such condition is like an engine without a governor, a ship without a rudder. Excess that is limited only by the extreme exhaustion of the physical forces can rarely be avoided. It is almost as sure to result as day is to follow night. And with this excess comes all sorts of weaknesses peculiar to woman. The man, too, feels exhausted, worn-out and debilitated most of the time. His physical energies, so seriously needed to carry on his business, or to assist him in reaching the goal of his ambitions, are all spent in excesses that never seem to end.

WOMAN'S DUTY TO POSSESS THIS INSTINCT.

Unquestionably man is much to be blamed for the usual unsatisfactory condition that follows most marriages, but it is the woman's duty to regulate sexual matters. She should possess a strongly defined instinct which should clearly indicate her actions. If she does not possess this instinct, she has not the slightest right to marry. And if possessed of this, and the husband refuses to be guided by it, they may just as well separate immediately, for no happiness will ever be found in marriage under such conditions.

That is the real, true cause of unhappiness in nearly all marriages. It causes that irritable, dissatified, feeling that makes quarreling so easily indulged. It is so hard for people to be honest, even to themselves, where sexual matters are concerned, but facts are facts and one cannot change them by any amount of prudish deceit.

DEGRADING INFLUENCE OF MARITAL MISERIES.

One can say much for happy marriages, much to encourage those who enter these sacred realms and find therein love, peace and happiness. But how about those who do not draw a prize?—those who are scorched in the fire of eternal discontent, who find that the bonds of matrimony goad the very soul, day after day, with stinging cruelty; that it animalizes the very best part of their nature, that it stifles every good and noble thought, that it crushes out every atom of wholesome ambition, and with the fangs of malicious hatred, created and fostered by this enforced unnatural relation, it poisons the very life of the principals in the tragedy. It matters not what the laws of man may be —the laws of justice, the laws of morality, the laws of nature, or even the laws of God, surely do not compel two poor victims of

matrimony to live together when it is an
actual sin against the higher laws of life,
when the deteriorating effects, physical and
mental, are as bad as if leading a fast life
with the lowest of human creatures. Marriage, if unhappy, depreciates the powers,
mental, physical and moral, and one had
a thousand times better remain single all
through life than to contract such an unsatisfactory union. It will take away all
hope, all ambition, everything that makes life
worth living. It will drag its victims down
the furthest extremes of misery and despair,
down to the lowest depths of human de-
pravity. The noblest character that ever
breathed could not resist the baneful influence of this condition of legalized prostitution. For what else can the enforced
relations of a loveless marriage be called?
When no love exists in this relation, there
remains only the lowest, the most bestial
passions. If the indulgence in these desires
is not prostitution, will some one please
define it?

Marry a woman in possession of a vigorous, wholesome, well-shaped body. Avoid

tight-laced waists as you would a scorpion, for though they may not sting you at the time, you may live to see the day when you will wish they had, for death is far preferable to life under some conditions, and one of these conditions is unquestionably that of being harried by marital miseries.

A MINISTER'S ARRAIGNMENT OF CORSETED WOMEN.

" Perhaps it is not putting it too strongly when we say that one-third of the great mass of young women are unqualified ever to become wives or mothers, because of false education and inherited or acquired infirmities. From one-half to two-thirds of all our married women suffer from some form of womb-trouble. Young girls, who are wholly ignorant of the delicate texture of their sexual organism, and without dreaming of the serious consequences which are to follow, contract their waists, and thus crowd the contents of the entire abdominal cavity below what is a natural position. By this means the womb is forced out of its designated place, and when the strain is continued, irritation and weakness result in a chronic condition, which quickly develops after marriage into the very prevalent 'falling of the womb,' causing a dragging or bearing-down sensation in the lower part of the abdomen, pain in the back, numbness of the lower limbs, and a general discomfort and misery, which must often be shared for years by all who dwell under the same roof with its unfortunate afflicted, unhappy, victim.

MARRIAGE A CURSE TO SUCH WOMEN.

" To a woman thus afflicted life is a burden, and marriage a curse, rather than a blessing. False ideas of form, cruel and destructive fashion and pernicious education, accomplish this terrible ruin of human life and human happiness. Cure, or even alleviation of discomfort and suffering, are doubtful and difficult, and the man who marries a woman with a compresssd waist may reasonably expect a sufficient inheritance of misery to last all the rest of his natural life. The man who marries such a woman, instead of obtaining a helpmate, imposes upon himself a burden. He may be ignorant of it at the time, but he will be sure to know it later on."—*Sylvanus Stall, D. D.*

Even if a girl possesses a vigorous body and strongly sexed nature, the corset pressing down on the delicate organs of sex, displaces and lessens the strength of the organs themselves, and every surrounding part.

That is the true reason why woman suffers so at childbirth. The abdomen and other muscles have been weakened, thus weakening the internal organs to a similar degree, and without that power so necessary under the circumstances, she naturally suffers seriously at this time.

Let the warning be plain. *Avoid corset-crushed waists, or prepare for marital miseries that will torture your soul like an animal that is being goaded with a red hot iron.*

Chapter XII.

SEXUAL ANNIHILATION OR STARVATION.

ERRONEOUS IMPRESSION OF SEXUAL NATURE

There is a ridiculous impression in the minds of some *prudes*, who have somehow acquired the idea that they are gifted with an excessive amount of refinement, that the sexual part of their nature is something vulgar, to be crushed out of mind and body. Unfortunately there are a few whose minds are so strong, or the sexual instincts so weak, that their efforts result in a sort of sexual annihilation or starvation. If they ever had any evidence of the possession of the magnetism and charm that nearly always accompany a person in a high degree of health, it disappears, and there remains a vacancy as it were. They even have a vacant expression which shows to the world their lack of sexual and general physical stamina, indicating, in reality, they are neither men **nor** women, but mere nonentities, from a sexual standpoint, and in nearly every **case** their abilities and powers in other directions **are** of a similar mediocre character.

MANLY MEN ALWAYS WELL SEXED.

In the same proportion that one succeeds in crushing out what he erroneously imagines to be his lower nature, to a similar degree will his powers in other ways deteriorate. A man to be of any importance must first *be a man*, and without that stamina, energy and general wholesome vigor, which is the usual accompaniment of finely sexed manhood, there is but small prospect of ever accomplishing anything of importance in life. Instead of adopting those means that will tend to lessen the powers of sex, it is the stern duty of every man to try to build and retain strength of this character. It makes him more manly, more courageous, capable of rising above the level of a mediocre existence.

GREATER STRENGTH MORE EASILY CONTROLLED.

There is not the slightest occasion for fear that one will acquire sexual strength which will grow beyond control. There is always greater strength of control under normal, than there is under abnormal conditions. Normal strength is steady, healthy—nothing unnatural or feverish about it; though very often under some momentary stimulus of feverish intensity even weak organs acquire an unnatural strength, which always react to their disadvantage by bringing about a relapse that often totally deprives them of power for a time.

CHAPTER XIII.

———

COMPLETE IMPOTENCE FROM OLD AGE AND OTHER CAUSES.

———

NERVOUS POWER CONTROLS SEXUAL STRENGTH.

As stated before, sexual power fluctuates as influenced by the nervous strength. It controls sexual strength, which is really an important part of the nervous organization. Therefore, anything that influences adversely the nervous organization has a similar influence on the sexual power.

If one neglects regular exercise—if no attention is given to those laws that are of such vast importance in the acquirement and retainment of vigorous health—regardless of how strong one may be from a sexual standpoint—he must expect his strength in this way gradually to decline, with a prospect of entire impotence. The effects of physical

decay are quickly manifested by the lessening of the sexual strength.

PREMATURE IMPOTENCE INDUCED.

Many men become impotent years and
years before such a result is necessary, for
the simple reason that they allow the general
physical health to decline in vigor, and fail
to make the necessary efforts to regain this
power, which really gives spice, enthusiasm
and zest to life.

This exhilaration, this excess of energy,
which shows itself in every vigorous man in
fine condition, is really nothing more than
the buoyant influence of abundant nervous
or sexual strength—both really mean the
same thing.   Wherever you find a man possesses one, he will always possess the other
to an equal degree.

Of course, all loss of sexual strength is
accompanied by general physical decline,
but men often lose power in this way, because
of their neglect in keeping their physical
forces to a normal standard of health, and
not because of any excess or other violations
of the laws of sex.

SEDENTARY HABITS CAUSE OF IMPOTENCE.

You can depend upon it as an unfailing rule that no man who follows strictly a sedentary occupation can for many years retain the virile powers of manhood. It is as certain to disappear as day is to follow night.

The normal circulation of the blood depends upon at least an occasional use of the entire muscular system. This use of the muscles disseminates the waste matter, and assists very materially in the work of elimination, thus all parts of the body are kept constantly in a superior condition.

A poor circulation and vigorous health are never co-existent. They do not go together. What is needed above all things in the development of sexual vigor is the perfect circulation of the blood throughout the entire body.

NO EXCUSE FOR LOSS OF THESE POWERS.

Of course, in early youth, when the vital forces are particularly strong, one may not conform to the laws of health in any way and still apparently possess all the vigor of superb vitality. But this will last only for a time   Premature loss of general health and sexual vigor will be influenced in time without the slightest doubt, just as sure as effect follows cause.

No man, regardless of age, has the slightest excuse for allowing his powers, in this way, to remain impotent.   As long as he is not actually a bed-ridden invalid, or is not suffering from some incurable chronic disease there is not the slightest excuse for either becoming or remaining impotent.

The sexual powers, given only a moderate amount of care, should last as long as life, and a man who allows this power to slip away has no one to blame but himself for his loss, and can blame no one but himself if he allows it to remain permanent.

We can promise a recovery and a strengthening of these powers with a certainty so absolute, so unfailing, that there remains not the slightest question if the sufferer accurately and regularly follows the rules we have laid down here for strengthening the nervous organism.

CHAPTER XIV.

———

UNDEVELOPED OR WASTED ORGANS.

———

HOW THESE DEFECTS CAN BE REMEDIED.

Where the sexual organ has wasted away from excesses and other debilitating influences, about the only remedy is to build up the nervous, digestive and muscular forces as advised here. Gradually your strength will return, and with this renewal of vigor, your sexual powers will very slowly appear. Of course the importance of these special exercises to strengthen and bring the blood to the adjacent muscles and organs cannot be emphasized too strongly. Cold bathing and plenty of fresh air allowed to come in direct contact with all parts of the body will be found of great value. A cure depends simply on your ability to bring back the nervous and muscular powers through the special system here illustrated.

A DANGEROUS REMEDY USEFUL IN RARE CASES ONLY.

Massage of the organ itself with an air pump, which is made for this particular purpose, will, no doubt, be of value in some special cases. This remedy is, however, very dangerous, and if used to excess may produce serious harm. It should be adopted only in extreme cases, and then should be used with utmost care to avoid any possible chance of excess. This device is a glass tube, somewhat larger than the average male organ, and is provided with a vacuum pump, which forces out the air. As the air is removed the blood is drawn down into the organ, gradually enlarging and drawing it out to its greatest possible size. The inventor claims that there is absolutely no sexual excitement connected with this—that it simply brings more blood to the organ, thus giving new life and vigor, as does a massage treatment when applied to the body.

In some few cases, where the sexual organ is unnaturally small, or where it has remained in an undeveloped state, this device will be of benefit, though it should not be used until all other means have failed—it should be the last resort.

The danger of over-stimulation of the organ when using a device of this character is very great, and its use should cease altogether when improvement is noted.

Any benefit derived from the use of this device, however, will be only transitory, if the means here advised for general physical improvement are not closely followed.

The device mentioned above will be forwarded by us on receipt of price, $6.00, though remember the writer's warning in reference to its use and the fact that it is of no value if the cause is simply depleted physical and nervous powers, and even when its use can be recommended it should be used only a few times with long intervals intervening. All letters referring to this, address to publishers and mark *personal.*

CHAPTER XV.

VARICOCELE.

SIMPLE REMEDY FOR THIS AGGRAVATING COMPLAINT.

This is usually the result of self-abuse in early life, though it often appears with excessive night losses. Sexual excess of almost any kind will cause it, however; as will also the weakening influences of any one of the various sexual diseases. Usually but little difficulty will be found in effecting a cure by very simple means. Of course, the general health should be made as vigorous as possible. The system of exercise as illustrated here should be taken regularly and all other advice followed that will evidently be beneficial. In addition to this the parts should be bathed twice per day, from two to five minutes, in very cold water. If a sitz bath can be taken, as advised in the chapter referring to bathing, recovery will be more rapid and certain. This appears to be a very simple means of cure, but unless an operation is absolutely essential it will effect the desired results in a very short time.

AVOID OLD EXCESSES.

It will be well to note, however, that if you go back to the old excesses, or if you allow yourself to decline in vigor, the trouble is liable to appear again. Avoid wearing any support for the scrotum unless absolutely necessary. A continued support is liable to weaken the walls of the scrotum, thus decreasing the strength of the testicles. A support under certain conditions is, no doubt, desirable, but it should be worn just as little as possible.

CHAPTER XVI.

———

METHODS OF TREATMENT.

———

DRUG TONICS OF ABSOLUTELY NO BENEFIT.

Let us emphasize at the very start that no drugs, no tonics of any kind. in form of electricity or belt of any description, can be of the slightest influence towards creating or strengthening sexual power. The remedy must come from within, must accompany the building up of all the physical forces. The circulation of the entire body must be awakened and brought up to a normal standard by natural means. Every sufferer from impotence has a poor circulation. These troubles are always co-existent.

Even if some stimulant can be found which will for a time arouse the organs of sex to renewed and abnormal activity, the ultimate result of this false stimulation will be to wear out the organs and bring on per-manent impotence just that much quicker.

NATURAL REMEDIES EFFECT RESULTS.

Nature! Depend on Nature and natural means entirely if you desire a cure. There is no excuse for impotence. One should retain the power of sex all through life, and if the laws of Nature have not been grossly violated, this can be done in every instance. If your powers in this way have been depleted or destroyed, rejuvenate them again by build-ing up the nervous and physical forces. The writer can promise with absolute certainty that this can be done in every case where the vitality of life still exists, if the natural methods described and illustrated in this book are adopted and carried out accurately and regularly for a sufficient length of time, though, as the powers begin to return, great care must be taken not to begin again the excess or unnatural drain which may have assisted in causing your condition.

Do not waste your time by trying this treatment for a few days only. Do not ex-pect any particularly noticeable change for at least two weeks, though very often decided improvement is noted in a few days.

INFALLIBLE METHODS HERE RECOMMENDED.

Do not for one minute allow yourself to doubt the ultimate satisfactory results of this treatment, for renewed sexual power is as absolutely certain if this method is followed as is the conclusion derived from a simple mathematical problem. These methods cannot fail. If enough strength is possessed to carry them out, you will have sufficient vitality to develop the desired results. Regardless of what your age or condition of health may be, unless you are actually a bed-ridden invalid, satisfactory results can be depended upon, for in nearly every case the principal cause of loss of this power is not sexual excess, but a general decline of the physical forces, and if these forces are built up—rejuvenated, as it were—and the circulation accelerated by natural means to the parts affected, thus increasing in vigor all the adjacent muscles and organs— the powers and vitality, in some cases almost equal to that of youth, return as a reward for the efforts made.

CAREFULLY PERUSE ALL INSTRUCTIONS.

Particular attention must be given to the instruction, and each chapter relating to the treatment must be carefully read and re-read, that the theory of the method may be thoroughly understood. An entire change will, no doubt, have to be made in your life, daily habits, diet, clothing, bathing, etc.; but lay aside your prejudices and give the methods as described a thorough trial. Many have labored under delusions in reference to diet and general habits of life, which have destroyed their strength of mind, body and sex, and ultimately their lives. Give these methods a fair trial. Give kindly Nature a chance to benefit you.

CHAPTER XVII.

SYSTEM OF EXERCISE FOR BUILD-ING VITAL AND SEXUAL POWER.

PROPER EXERCISE PRODUCES NORMAL HEALTH.

Muscular exercise, adapted to the needs of the individual, tends to produce, in every case, a more normal condition. For instance, if one is too fleshy to be in normal health, it will take off flesh; if too thin, it will add flesh. This ability of physical culture to bring about the highest degree of normal health is exemplified with equal emphasis in sexual life. Those who suffer from weakness in this way will find in specially adapted train-ing the only safe means of cure. As the muscles develop, the digestive power in-creases, the circulation improves, the nerves are strengthened, and the mind freshened with renewed confidence. This building up of the physical strength affects beneficially every organ of the body. The same can be said of its effects on those suffering sexually from an excess of animal life. This is a disease just the same as the other extreme, and this surplus energy can be absorbed and used to advantage if expended in muscular exercise. Not only does the muscle and nerve power increase, and the general health vastly improve when this method is followed, but the unusual and unnatural strength of this abnormal desire disappears, creating in reality a greater, safer strength, and removing the feverishness of an over-wrought nervousness.

INACTIVE MUSCLES SLOWLY DEGENERATE.

Activity is the law of life   Inactivity means decay. Long-continued stagnation means death. Some men have the incomprehensible audacity to believe that their muscular system can remain idle indefinitely without losing in the slightest degree that symmetry and strength they have acquired through extreme activity in early life. They seem to forget that an inactive muscle slowly degenerates, grows smaller and weaker and gradually lessens in firmness and symmetry. The lesson so plainly taught of the wasting away of an unused muscle when a bone has been broken should be remembered. The first time an opportunity is secured, examine the muscle on a broken arm after it has had a complete rest of a few weeks. You will find it wasted almost to nothing. There is no more startling example of the results of muscular inactivity than this. The entire muscular system will waste away to a similar degree if it does not receive regular use, and it is not entirely this wasting process that is to be deplored—the general vigor of the body is lessened to a similar degree. The nervous organism is weakened in exactly the same proportion, and with this nervous degeneracy, of course, comes the decay of the sexual powers.

MUSCLE REPLACED BY FATTY TISSUE.

To be sure, if you are leading an inactive life, you may not notice this wasting process, for if the digestive powers are good, as the muscles disappear fatty tissue will be deposited to replace them. Thus externally you see but little change, though there will be a tremendous change in strength. For a moment the strength may seem almost as great as ever, but when continued efforts, even for a short time, are required, the loss of muscular power is readily detected.

UTILITY OF SEXUAL POWERS GOVERNS THEIR LIFE.

Let the writer emphasize the statement that impotence always ultimately follows long-continued muscular inactivity. This result is as certain to appear as day is to follow night. It is the law of Nature that it should be so. The sexual powers of man were given for the perpetuation of his kind. When his powers so decline that he possesses nothing worth transmitting, then the power of reproduction, and often all sexual desire, is removed. Utility is the law of the universe. When anything or any power ceases to be useful it disappears.

EXERCISE ACCELERATES CIRCULATION TO ALL PARTS.

The effect of cultivating sexual vigor by building up the muscular and vital powers of the body can not be fittingly described. If all powers in this way are lost, or if they seem to have so diminished in vigor that the intense desire of vigorous pulsating youth has disappeared, they can be entirely regained by natural processes assisted by the muscular movements here described; since the bringing of rich blood in copious quantities to every part of the body which results from these exercises is one of the salient features necessary in order to regain the sexual powers.

Under the influence of proper exercise for every muscle of the body, the heart, with quick and strong and greatly accelerated pulsations, forces the blood with increased power through the arteries and capillaries, drives the impurities out through the great purifying organs, the skin and kidneys, and causes every organ of the body to be rejuvenated and strengthened.

EXERCISE AN INTERNAL CLEANSING AGENT.

The effects of exercise can be fitly compared to a bath. It cleanses the internal system just as hot water and soap cleanses the external.   The vast nervous organism, with branches reaching throughout the most minute parts of the body, feels the great benefit of this internal cleansing process almost immediately.   As the muscles grow stronger, firmer and more symmetrical, the power and delicacy of the nervous system vastly increase, and like a guitar string that is toned up just to the right pitch, every nerve will quickly respond when required with the harmony of exquisite, delightful music.   No cigar smoker or whiskey drinker ever tasted in all its fulness, the marvelous intensity and power, of full, complete, sexual strength. Benumbed nerves cannot feel; perverted emotions cannot produce that which is competely satisfying.   Something is always wanting.

ANY SYSTEM USING ALL THE MUSCLES BENEFICIAL.

Any ordinary system of exercise that uses to a moderate degree all the muscles of the body will, of course, be found beneficial in accelerating the circulation and increasing the virile powers of man; but those movements that are especially advantageous

for strengthening the vigor of those parts of
the body closely surrounding the organs of
sex will be found vastly more valuable in
speedily producing the desired results. The
exercise of these muscles accelerates the
circulation directly to those parts, and naturally the benefit which accrues to them, by
the renewed life brought in the quickened
circulation, is shared by the sexual organs
also. Thus, in selecting a system of muscular exercise especially for strengthening
and for bringing into life dormant sexual
powers, the writer has devised a series of
movements that strengthen not only the
lungs, heart and organs of digestion and
general vital system, but directly affect the
sexual organs by vastly increasing the supply of new, rich blood to all the surrounding parts.

REGULATE EXERCISE ACCORDING TO STRENGTH.

The amount of exercise that should be
taken by each individual at the start must
be determined entirely by the strength possessed. Continue each movement until a

verv slight feeling of fatigue ensues. Rest a moment only, and then go on to the next exercise. Be very careful not to exercise too much at first.

Take each movement say five or eight times at the start. Increase one or two each day, and after having practiced daily for ten days or two weeks, each one can then be continued until you are tired.

The exercise should be taken while lying in bed, immediately on awakening.

Your room should, of course, be thoroughly supplied with fresh air by proper ventilation at all times, but especial care must be used to see that there is a plentiful supply of pure air when taking these exercises.

PURE AIR OF GREAT IMPORTANCE.

Open the windows wide.

When thoroughly awake throw the covers off. If especially cold, a few of the exercises can be taken to warm the body, before throwing off the covers, though it will be found of especial advantage for you to follow the advice given in a preceding chapter and accustom yourself gradually to cold air. But there is no need of exposing yourself too much at the start.

Be very moderate in any change you intend to make.

As soon as you are inured to the cold air, instead of merely throwing off the covers, you should, in addition, remove every particle of clothing, so that you can take your exercise entirely nude, as previously advised, but do not try this at first.

The writer repeats: *Be Moderate!* Feel your way, step by step! How do you know but that this treatment may be another fake?

BE BORN AGAIN.

When a man sees and feels that he can practically be born over again, that he can be made almost like new, by a few systematic, sensible efforts; if there is a spark of vitality within him, he will immediately endeavor to secure the rewards so easily within his reach.

If you have had the usual experience, you have no doubt spent large sums of money and still larger quantities of time in searching for the remedy that we offer you here practically for nothing. Give the methods here advised a trial for two weeks, and after that there will be no need to spur you on to further efforts—you will continue without the necessity of such incentives.

If you feel tired before going through all the movements advised, do not try to finish them the first few times. At the conclusion of your reclining exercises, stand on the floor and take an exercise similar to jumping a rope until you begin to breathe freely, then draw in a few deep inhalations, after which take a cold sitz bath (immersing hips only in water.) If this cannot be done conveniently, take a cold sponge bath, and stoop down over a basin of water, dipping up the water and allowing it to run freely over the private organs.

After the covers are removed you can begin the exercises, bearing in mind the instructions given in reference to how long each movement should be continued.

Exercise No. 1.—Recline flat on back. raise the hips as high as you can off the bed, the weight, of course, resting on heels and

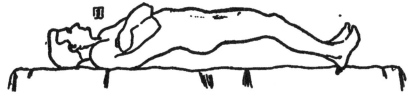

shoulders. For muscles on posterior portion of hips and small of back.

Exercise No. 2.—Recline on right side. Now raise the hips (knees straight) as high as you can from the bed, the weight resting

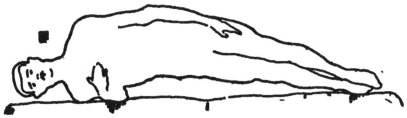

on right foot and right arm and shoulder. The same exercise reclining on left side. For muscles on sides from waist to thighs.

Exercise No. 3—Recline on the back and

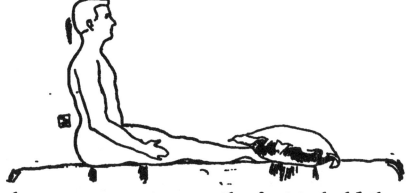

place some covers over the feet to hold them

down. Now, with hands placed on thighs, raise to a sitting position without assisting with the hands. For the muscles of the abdomen.

Exercise No. 4.—Recline on the stomach. Grasp the head of the bed somewhere tightly with the hands. Now, without

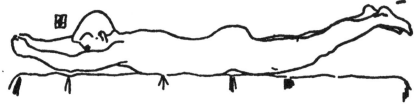

bending the knees, raise both legs as high as possible. Not very much of a movement can be made in this exercise, but it is valuable for affecting the muscles of small of back, and large muscles on posterior portion of hips.

Exercise No. 5.—Recline on back. Now

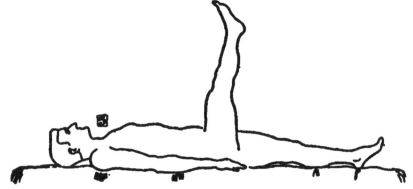

raise right leg with knee straight until as

illustrated.   Same exercise with left leg.
For muscles of anterior portion of upper
thighs.

Exercise No. 6.—Recline on right side.
Now raise left leg with knee straight as

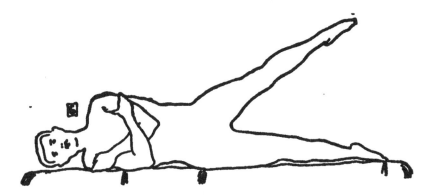

high as you · can upward.   Same exercise
with right leg while reclining on left side.
For outer portion of upper thighs.

Exercise No. 7.—Recline on back.   Now
bring right leg with knee straight as far as

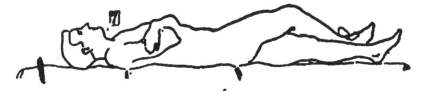

possible over left leg.   Same exercise with
right leg.   For muscles on inside of upper
thighs.

Exercise No. 8.—Recline on stomach.
Now raise right leg with knee straight as

far upward as possible. Same exercise with

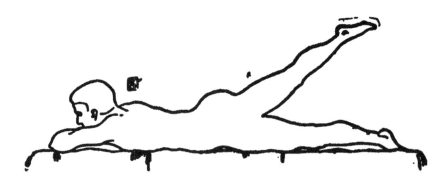

left leg. For muscles on posterior portion of hips.

Exercise No. 9.—Recline on back. Now grasp hold of something behind the head,

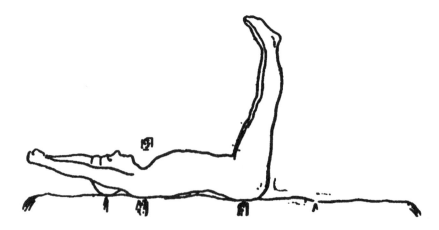

then raise both feet as high as you can. For muscles of lower part of abdomen and upper part of tighs.

Exercise No. 10.—Recline on back. Now bend both knees as much as possible, then kick out straight upward with right and left

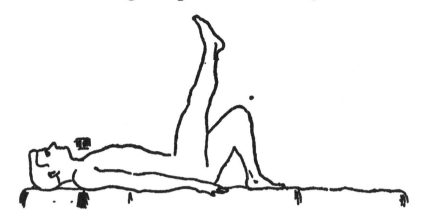

legs alternately. For muscles in central portion of upper leg.

Exercise No. 11.—Recline on right side. Now cross right leg at ankle over left leg just above knee, then raise the hips as high

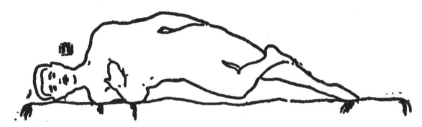

as you can, the weight resting on right shoulder and left leg. Same exercise reclining on left side. For muscles on inside of thighs and lateral portion of waist.

Exercise No. 12.—Recline on stomach. Now cross the right ankle over the left ankle, then bend the left leg at knee as much as possible, raising the weight of lower right leg. Same exercise with right

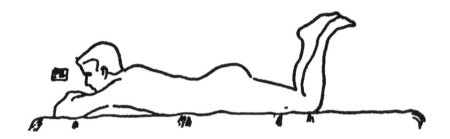

leg. For muscles of the posterior portion of central upper leg.

Chapter XVIII.

SPECIAL COURSE OF EXERCISES.

ESPECIALLY FOR DEVELOPING CHEST, SHOULDERS, BACK AND ARMS.

The course here illustrated is to be added to the reclining exercises after you have become inured to the work, say in ten days or two weeks. Continue to take the morning exercise as advised, but take this course just before retiring in the evening.

Do not forget the necessity of fresh, pure air, and see that the windows are wide open.

Continue each movement until slightly tired.

If you have an exerciser, or are following some good system of exercise similar to that of the writer's with device made for that particular purpose, there will be no necessity for taking these movements. The course with the apparatus can take its place.

Don't forget that the less clothes worn

during the exercise the better. Exercise vigorously, put vim, life, energy, determination in every movement, every effort.

Exercise No. 1.—Assume position as per Fig. 1. Hold elbows at sides, and raise hands up and down quickly forty to sixty times. Now draw in full breath, all you can, and hold it while you make twenty move-

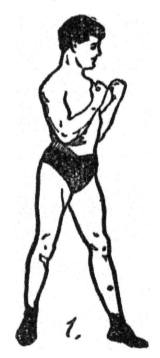

ments. Repeat three times. Now flex the muscles of arms, and imagine you are lifting a very heavy weight, and bring hands up and down very slowly. This is for developing the arms.

Exercise No. 2.—Assume position as per illustration No. 2. Draw in deep inspiration, all you can. Now hold this breath, and, keeping elbows rigid, swing arms quick and

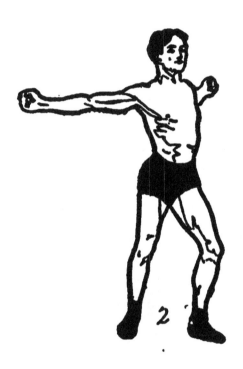

strong, far backward and forward on a level with shoulders as long as you can conveniently retain the breath. Repeat until tired. For expanding the chest and increasing lung power.

Exercise No. 3.—Stand erect, with feet far

apart.   Now touch the floor far to the right,

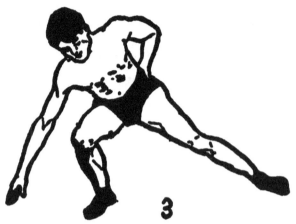

3

as per illustration; then far to the left.   Repeat exercise from ten to twenty times.

Exercise No. 4.—Assume position as per illustration No. 4.   Keep knees very rigid, raise hands high as you can over head with

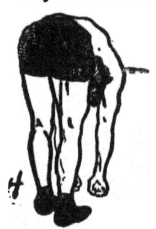

elbows rigid, from fifteen to twenty-five times.   For strengthening the back.

Exercise No. 5.—Strongly brace yourself as per illustration No. 5.   Now strike out hard and quick with right and left hands alternately, reaching out as· far as you can at each blow. Continue until tired. Count each time, to see how you are able to improve in endurance.

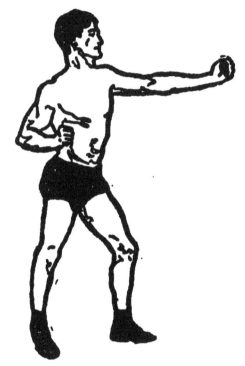

Complete your evening exercise by taking ten full, deep breaths before an open window. Throw shoulders far back and hold each breath about twenty seconds. Always breathe through the nose.

Sometime during the day (not immediately after a hearty meal) walk about two miles at a fast gait, increase this walk a quarter of a mile each day until you are walking six miles per day. During this walk draw in many deep breaths, occasionally retain breath for a moment, drawing shoulders up and back as far as you can and holding them in this position. While holding the shoulders in this position contract the muscles of the arms and chest as tensely as possible.

Conclude each time with a jumping exercise similar to jumping a rope, and, if strong enough, jump back and forth over some obstacle.

Do not forget to take a hot bath, with plenty of soap and water, two or three times per week after evening exercise.

Chapter XIX.

—

THE WALK TONIC.

—

HEALTH CAN BE SECURED FROM WALKING.

The great physical benefit that can be derived from walking will actually astound anyone who will give it a thorough trial. Not walking as ordinarily understood, but walking for pleasure, for health.

No matter what sort of a contest an athlete may be training for, walking always constitutes an important part of the work. All trainers claim it hardens and develops the muscles and gives great endurance.

The walk must be taken with a different spirit from that which usually exists under such circumstances. Put energy, life, action in every movement, every impulse.

LET THE OBJECT OF WALKING BE HEALTH.

Walk as though it was a pleasure, and if you are serious in your attempts, the result will be thorough enjoyment of the exercise. As to the distance necessary to produce the best results, the writer advises that the walk be continued until there is a feeling of fatigue, until a comfortable seat is enjoyed. Never, under any circumstances, become too ambitious at first. It is far better to lean toward the side of moderation.

Gradually increase the distance as you become thoroughly familiar with your strength and requirements.

Now come the important instructions in reference to this walk if the greatest benefits are to be derived.

GIVE CAREFUL ATTENTION TO THIS.

For a short distance you must walk rather slowly. Gradually increase until you are traveling at a gait considered fast for you. As speed is increased begin to inhale deeply, always through the nose, expanding the chest to its greatest capacity. At each time the lungs are completely filled, retain the breath for a short time, flex (make tense and hard) the muscles of the arms and chest, bring the shoulders far back and draw the abdomen in. Hold the shoulders in this position for a short time, and make several endeavors to bring them still farther back. This exercise will tend to give proper carriage, and in connection with the special breathing, will cause you to realize that it is really and truly a " walk tonic."

CHAPTER XX.

DIET.

IMPORTANCE OF PROPER FOODS.

No matter what precautions may be taken with the object of building a higher degree of physical health, unless you are following a wholesome nourishing diet but little or no improvement can be acquired. In fact, nothing indicates the importance of a properly arranged diet so clearly as the fact that some people have actually kept in health by careful attention to the quantity and character of the foods used, giving but little attention to exercise.

IN REFERENCE TO VEGETARIANISM.

Although the writer favors a vegetarian diet, he eats just what his appetite craves, and if meat is desired, which often occurs, he does not refuse to satisfy this demand. In fact, unless one is living at an institution where the various varieties of vegetarian foods can be secured, properly prepared, or unless you have the essential knowledge in securing this variety and can prepare or have these various foods prepared, vegetarianism had better be strictly avoided. Many have lessened their physical power quite materially by endeavoring to follow certain diets without the knowledge or ingredients necessary. Any change in diet should be slowly adopted. Do not stop suddenly eating foods that have apparently agreed with you and start immediately on an entirely different regimen. Feel your way, step by step on any new diet you may choose to adopt.

READ BOOKS ON DIET.

Diet is really a study in itself, and if the reader desires thorough familiarity with the subject, the writer would advise that he read several of the very valuable books that treat of it. Do not read one only, and take that as a standard. Read several, and draw your own conclusions. In this way your knowledge of diet becomes a part of you, and there is no necessity for referring to some book when desirous of securing some particular information.

POWER OF THE IMAGINATION.

The statement is often quoted that " What is one man's food, is another man's poison." This is not true, though in many false statements one may find a grain of truth, and it is so with this.   Everyone knows the great power of the imagination over the body. It has an equal power over the stomach and digestive forces generally. If one eats a food that he believes is harmful, he is continually searching with all the keenness of his imagination for signs to indicate that the expected trouble has actually begun, and in this way so centres his attention to that organ that the expected symptoms are really produced.

Disguise any wholesome, nourishing food which the appetite craves, and which is supposed to result in injury, and have a person eat it under the supposition that it is something else, and in nearly every case the painful symptoms experienced before whenever the food was eaten will not appear.

DEVELOP A NORMAL APPETITE.

Of course, we must admit that the digestive powers of various individuals differ very
greatly, and although one may be able to ex-
tract the desired nourishment from a certain
article of food, another may have some defect in his digestive organs, or the gastric
juices, which will make it difficult to use this
food to advantage; therefore the importance
of developing and depending on a normal
appetite to select a satisfactory diet cannot
be too strongly emphasized. A normal appetite craves most strongly that special food
element which is needed the most at that
particular time to nourish the body. Most
appetites are normal until made morbid by
overeating, eating when not hungry, and
other weakening practices. The craving
for unwholesome foods in nearly every case
indicates that the stomach has become injured by stuffing, and the mass of fermented
food with which it is struggling often creates
an appetite for almost anything that will
assist in bringing relief. The appetite for
alcoholic stimulants, for instance, is always
greatly increased if the stomach is suffering

from overeating or from a series of meals eaten without appetite.

GLADSTONE'S RULE FOR MASTICATION.

Nearly every authority on diet will advise one to eat slowly, but that does not mean to chew slowly. You can move your jaws as fast as desired. In fact, the faster one chews the more copiously the saliva flows, and consequently the more quickly the food is ready to be swallowed.

Gladstone is reported to have said that each mouthful of food should be chewed thirty times, and this calculation is very nearly correct if one desires the saliva to play its important part in the digestive process.

FOOD MUST BE ENJOYED.

Chew your food thoroughly. Get all the enjoyment out of the process of eating that you possibly can. It is an actual sin against your own body to eat without hunger. One of the most important digestive processes is brought into thorough action by the keen enjoyment of food. It is not only the saliva but the gastric juice of the stomach that flows more freely when food is intensely enjoyed. But if no hunger is experienced when eating—if the food is washing down without appetite or enjoyment—the digestive process is carried on with great difficulty, and no one can enjoy vigorous health under such circumstances. Food eaten under such conditions is of absolutely no benefit. It had far better not be eaten at all. It simply gives the digestive organs that much more of a load to eliminate. No strength is gained from it. It really lessens the muscular strength, for it takes the blood away from the muscles, that it may assist in the process of ridding the digestive organs of the additional load that has been introduced without excuse.

FOOD EATEN WITHOUT HUNGER LESSENS STRENGTH.

But you may say, "I must keep up my strength. I seem to be growing weaker all the time, and must eat, or I won't be able to walk." The very means you have adopted to keep up your strength is the actual cause of your weakness.

Wait for an appetite if not hungry. Let this be an unfailing rule. You cannot possibly enjoy vigorous health if this rule is not recognized and followed.

HOW HUNGER CAN BE CULTIVATED.

But some will say, "Why, I would never grow hungry."

You need not worry one moment about this. Fast from one to seven days, and there will not be the slightest doubt that your appetite will be resurrected in all its youthful intensity, and with this appetite will come renewed enjoyment of everything in life. Food will then benefit you. It will be digested, and new life, new energy will thrill your nerves when this new, rich blood begins to circulate.

If the diet is confined to foods that possess the elements of nourishment, it is not so much a question of what one eats, as how much is eaten.

Eat what you can digest—what your appetite calls for—not all you can stuff into your stomach.

When the food palls—when it ceases to be

eaten with a keen relish—stop right there! Do not eat another bite.

SUPERFINE WHITE FLOUR NOT A FOOD.

Avoid white flour and all articles of food made from it. No food for muscles, brain, or bones can be extracted from superfine flour. All these important food elements have been removed with the bran. Not only is white flour greatly defective in all nourishing qualities, but in numerous cases it is the actual cause of constipation. (Note chapter on Constipation.) Eat whole wheat bread instead of white bread whenever you can get it. Whole wheat flour is just what its name implies. It is made from the whole grain of wheat. No bran or any part has been extracted. It is really a perfect food when eaten thus, for it contains in almost exact proportions the food elements necessary to properly nourish the body. See that this whole wheat flour is used instead of the white in every food requiring flour. You will find that this will make a great difference in your general condition almost at once You will feel better nourished, more energetic.

Cultivate an appetite for acid fruits. They can be especially recommended at all times.

Eat wholesome, nourishing foods, and avoid all fancy, highly-seasoned dishes.

TWO MEALS EACH DAY ADVISED.

If you experiment with your diet somewhat you will, no doubt, find that two meals per day will agree with you better than three. You may not be aware that when the stomach is overworked the digestive juices are not supplied in proper quantities, and the result is the food seems to create no strength, no energy. This is caused by overeating or eating too often. The remedy is to eat less often and thus give the stomach a rest and allow it to store up gastric juice for the next meal.

Whole wheat bread, eggs, salads with oil dressing and nourishing vegetables can be especially commended in building up the virile powers. Good fresh meats, when especially craved and easily digested, are also useful, though it is usually well to avoid immature meats, such as veal, lamb and the like.

Do not fail to keep in mind the necessity for the thorough enjoyment of food. Eat that which you keenly relish, and leave all articles of food strictly alone if not relished.

In numerous cases fasting for a few meals, or even for several days, will be found of great value in bringing about a normal condition, though before attempting a long fast it would be well to make sure of your position. "Be sure you are right, then go ahead."

Chapter XXI.

BATHING.

IMPORTANCE OF A CLEAN SKIN.

A clean skin is positively necessary to the enjoyment of the highest degree of health. Not because dirt is particularly injurious to the body, but because it clogs up the pores and lessens their activity, thus retaining impurities or sending them to find other means for elimination.

A writer of some reputation on one occasion maintained that the benefits of daily bathing was generally exaggerated. He stated truly that the skin was made up of millions of tiny scales that overlap each other like shingles on a roof top, and that as one scale was worn out, it was discarded and a new one was underneath to take its place, and he claimed that an undue amount of bathing loosened these scales prematurely, exposing the new scales before being sufficiently hardened. He also stated that the too frequent use of soap and hot water absorbed the natural oil of the skin, and had a tendency to make it dry and harsh.

HOW THE BODY CLEANS ITSELF.

There is unquestionably some truth in this writer's remarks, especially in his statement in reference to the too frequent use of hot water and soap. A hot bath should not be taken over two or three times per week. Some writers claim that a daily hot bath is necessary to cleanliness.

This writer's assertion that the body cleans itself by casting off scales as they become dried is true, and if the body were exposed to the air to the same extent as that of any ordinary animal, one would not suffer very much if he never took a bath, though it would be well to note that many of the animals and birds find enjoyment in occasional baths if there occurs an opportunity for taking them. It is the clothing which shuts out the air and which absorbs the impurities cast off from the body that makes frequent bathing so necessary. The activity of the pores of the skin is absolutely necessary to the acquirement of the highest degree of health. The importance of this cannot be overestimated. The writer was informed on one occasion by one who formerly suffered a great deal from rheumatic pains that he entirely removed the trouble by daily accelerating the action of the pores with aid of two soft bristle brushes which he used all over his body.

EXCESS POSSIBLE IN ANYTHING.

Unquestionably one can bathe too much. One can eat too much bread. Exercise can be taken too much. In fact, no matter how beneficial anything may be, it can be the means of producing injury if excess is allowed.

Though it is certainly possible to bathe too much, the writer believes there is but little danger of this in any case.

The accumulation of the perspiration and other impure matter eliminated through the pores makes a hot bath with plenty of soap necessary at least two or three times per week.

GREAT BENEFIT OF FRICTION BATHS.

While treating yourself for sexual weaknesses of any kind the morning exercise should always be followed by a friction bath. This bath is taken by brushing the skin all over with two soft bristle brushes. Use the brushes back and forth over every part of the skin until it is pink from the accelerated circulation brought to the surface by the friction.

The skin will naturally be very tender in the beginning, though it will soon become inured, and the brushes can be used for a considerable time with each treatment.

The effect of this friction bath on the appearance of the skin is wonderful. In a short time it will become as smooth and soft as velvet, and absolutely free from all pimples and blotches, if a rational system of diet is being followed.

This friction bath should be followed immediately by a cold sitz bath, of about one minute's duration. A sitz bath is the immersion of the hips only in water, and it can be taken more conveniently in a tub made for the purpose. A small tub, or an ordinary washtub will serve, or a large bathtub will do if one is agile enough to place the heels on the end and then lower the body in the water, allowing the feet to remain as placed. After sitting in the water about one minute, wet the body all over and dry quickly with a rough towel.

If there are no conveniences for taking this sitz bath wet the body all over with cold water, and stoop down over a basin until you can easily bath the private parts in this cold water.

EASILY TO BECOME INURED TO COLD WATER.

The friction bath may be discontinued after recovery, but it will be found a powerful tonic in aiding the system to retain normal vigor, and should by no means be neglected.

Many shrink from the use of cold water, and believe that they cannot become accustomed to it. This can easily be done without any shock worth mentioning if the proper process is adopted. Gradually accustom yourself to it. Make the water a little colder each day. Many, however, find not the slightest difficulty in taking cold baths right from the first when they follow immediately after the exercises and friction bath. The circulation is so awakened by these influences that the body is sufficiently able to resist the shock, and the after effects are exceedingly pleasant.

If cold after a cold bath always exercise until warm. This will insure against any possibility of ill-effects.

IMPORTANCE OF ACTIVITY OF THE PORES.

Do not forget that if the entire surface of the body was varnished over, death would ensue in a few hours, because of the accumulation of impurities that usually find their outlet through the pores. Nothing could prove the absolute necessity for regular bathing more emphatically than this one fact. Of course, there are many who bathe only on rare occasions, and a few who never bathe at all, but they are the kind who are satisfied with merely existing. They do not live in the true sense of the word. In order to live, in order to feel the energy and power of superb health, pulsating in your every nerve, your every muscle—in order to be thrilled with the power of life and health and joy, every physical function must be in perfect working order, and this cannot be possible unless the pores of the skin are kept cleaned and active by regular bathing.

CHAPTER XXII.

IMPORTANCE OF PURE AIR.

AIR IS A FOOD.

Pure air is absolutely essential to life, to health. One can exist on bad air, but to exist does not necessarily mean living. Air usually seems to be of little importance. The average individual imagines that it has but little influence on his general health. There was never a more serious blunder. There is food in air. Oxygen is a food. It is just as necessary, in fact far more necessary, to life than any other element which enters into the constituents of the body. A man can live for sixty days without solid food; he can live for several days without water, but he can not live for five minutes without oxygen. Did you ever think of that? Consider the importance and enormous value of pure air, rich in this oxygen that the lungs may be liberally supplied with their needs. You cannot acquire or retain sexual or any kind of power for any length of time if this necessity for pure air is not recognized.

SUPERSTITIOUS FEAR OF DRAUGHTS.

Are you afraid of draughts? Well hurry up and rid yourself of this ridiculous fear. This has "dug" premature graves for thousands. Did you ever notice that the more a man feared draughts the more colds he seemed to acquire, the weaker he seemed to be, while the careless man who gave but little attention to that which is supposed to be essential for various cold seasons of the years, was stronger, and rarely, if ever, had a cold? The latter was stronger because his lungs were fed with a plentiful supply of oxygen at all times, and the thousands of little pores all over his body also had a chance to breathe.

Do not waste your time by taking any of the treatment advised here unless you can at once make up your mind to feed the lungs and every part of the body with oxy.

gen. Do not sleep in a badly ventilated room. Open the windows wide—the wider the better. Cultivate a love for fresh air. Breathe it deeply at all times; bathe your body in it. It means life, health, strength. It is the greatest tonic in the world. It absorbs the impurities that are thrown off from the body and assists greatly in accelerating the process of elimination constantly going on through the pores.

DELICATE PLANT COMPARED TO A WEAK BODY.

Of course, if accustomed to smothering yourself with clothing, do not immediately adopt the other extreme. Your body is like a plant made delicate by being kept from sun and air. If such a plant is immediately exposed to rough breezes and the direct rays of the sun, it is liable to suffer from this sudden change, but expose it a short time the first day, a little more the next day, gradually increasing each day, and finally it will become vigorous and hardy, capable of bearing any amount of exposure. A weak body is exactly like this plant. No more suitable comparison could be made. By coddling and extreme care, breathing the vile atmosphere of inclosed rooms over and over again, until actually rotten with the poisons emanating from the lungs, and by fear of all draughts and sunlight, one can easily deteriorate into a fragile plant, and will remain delicate and weak as long as that which creates this condition is allowed to exist.

RIGHT ABOUT, FACE!

Turn over a new leaf at once. Pure air—not rotten air—was made to breathe! Inclosed air becomes rotten, foul, disease-breeding.

BENEFITS OF AIR BATHS.

The only way that cold air ever injured anyone was when it had frozen a part of his body.

The writer takes an air bath daily. It is necessary to the acquirement and retainment of a highest degree of health. Take your exercise in your own room nude, with the windows open, and open them wider each day. Build the internal fire! Make the blood warm your body while in this nude state by vigorous movements.

The writer follows this practice in the coldest of weather. Often when the thermometer registered below zero he has exercised nude in his room with the windows wide open and with the wind blowing full upon him. Strange as this may seem to the average reader, this exercise in such cold atmosphere is most thoroughly enjoyed after a few movements have been made. Of course, when first coming from a warm bed one feels cold; but this passes away in a short time and there follows a feeling of exhilaration, or physical exaltation, which is hard to describe.

COLD AIR A GREAT TONIC.

The more colds are feared and the more attempts made to protect yourself against them by coddling, the more colds you will acquire. This is an unfailing rule, and no one who gives the matter any attention can question its truth. The direct contact of the skin with air influences greater activity of the pores; this is occasioned because the circulation has been accelerated to the surface. Air baths have a most wonderfully beneficial effect in this way, and the importance of allowing the surface of the body to come in direct contact with the air as much as possible cannot be too strongly emphasized. It will be a valuable means of assisting in the building of a vigorous, healthy nervous and muscular organism, though it is especially beneficial to the nervous system, having a quieting and strengthening effect on the entire nervous organism.

Begin at once to cultivate a love for fresh pure air. It will almost immediately begin to increase the virile powers of manhood, and you will reap rewards from a habit of this kind that could not be purchased in any other way by all the wealth in Christendom.

CHAPTER XXIII.

———

MENTAL INFLUENCE.

———

GREAT POWER OF MIND OVER BODY.

We have already mentioned the power of mental influence over the body under certain conditions, and in fact it possesses a great influence in any condition of health or disease. In suggestive therapeutics and in Christian science, we find this influence given first place as a remedial agency, and they have built an elaborate system of treatment which apparently depends entirely on the faith of the patient. This is magnifying the power of mind over body unquestionably, but the importance of this must not be overlooked.

Thousands of healthy human beings go about with a dread on their mind that they are suffering from some insiduous disease, when their ailment really exists only in their imagination. Such a condition, if continued long, will, however, produce actual disease, and this mental condition must be discouraged as much as possible. Remember that disease or weakness is unnatural, and that the body, if given an opportunity, will actually cure itself, and no matter how serious may be your trouble, vow that you will make the necessary efforts to secure health, and that you do not merely hope to secure it, but that you intend to see that you do one way or another. Use your will power. Put out of mind any thought or suggestion that any other results than those desired can possibly appear, and you will be amazed at the influence this will have toward bringing about recovery.

HAVE AN OBJECT! BE SOMEBODY!

"Every young man who desires to remain strong, or to regain his physical, intellectual and moral powers, should have an absorbing purpose in life. Live with an aim, and let that aim be high. The man who aims at the sun will shoot higher than the man who aims at the earth. If you do not build a few castles in the air, you never will own any that are built on the earth. Devote yourself with untiring diligence to some department of work. Determine what is to be your life-purpose, and devote yourself absorbingly to its attainment. Do not be contented with mediocrity. Rise above the masses. Attain to eminence. Be thorough from the very be-ginning. Be diligent. And if you will thus devote yourself to the untiring attainment of some worthy purpose, there can be no question in regard to your future acquisition, your life will be worth something."—*Sylvanus Stall, D.D.*

GLOOMY THOUGHTS ARE ENEMIES.

This influence of mind over body is of especial importance in all sexual troubles. Ailments of this nature seem to cast a gloom over the victim that is difficult to dissipate. But do not allow it to encompass you! Fight it as you would an enemy, for it is an enemy and should be treated as such, Keep it as far away as possible. Be pleasant with your-self. Make yourself good company for your-self and for others. Cultivate a smiling

ountenance.   If your features are growing
into a chronic, worried expression, command
them to smile occasionally.   Think of something funny as often as possible.   Look at
the humorous side of life.   The best time to
joke is when death stares you in the face.
Anyway, why fear death?   You only have
to die once.   It usually takes more courage
to live than it does to die.   Anybody can die!
That is simple; but there are occasions when
it takes real bravery and determination to
live.

DO YOUR BEST, THEN STOP BOTHERING.

Let your first efforts toward building the
virile powers of superb manhood be spent in
endeavoring to cultivate a cheerful countenance.   Stop worrying at once.   It is a waste
of vital strength—it is a strain on nerves and
muscles—it keeps you in a tense, rigid condition as though you were constantly on the
alert for fear of some terrible calamity.   Do
the best you can, and then say to yourself:
I don't care what happens.   I've done my
best.   I'm not at fault."

The most severe criticism is where you have a complaint to make against yourself. One can stand the criticism of others, but self-blame is the most cutting of all to a conscientious person, Therefore, see that you have no cause for self-blame, and then stop bothering.

CHAPTER XXIV.

CONSTIPATION.

INJURIOUS EFFECTS OF THIS TROUBLE.

If habitually constipated, any sexual trouble that may exist is seriously aggravated, and effective means should be adopted immediately on commencing treatment to remedy any tendency in this direction. Usually the adoption of a satisfactory diet and the daily use of the exercises recommended, will prove an effective remedy, but in case it does not, more harsh methods must be used for a time. Do not depend on purgative drugs under any circumstances. This will really make the trouble far more serious in character and ultimately render a cure much more difficult to reach.

FOODS RECOMMENDED.

Cultivate an appetite for all acid fruits, such as oranges, apples, pears, cherries, strawberries, blackberries, etc. Avoid white flour as you would a poison. Many suffer seriously with this ailment from this one article of diet. Superfine white flour has a most seriously binding influence on the bowels, no matter in what form it may be eaten—in bread, biscuit or pastry. Eat whole-wheat bread when you can get it, and, if possible, have all articles of food requiring flour made with whole-wheat flour (See chapter on Diet for reason). If your are careful not to eat too fast and also not to over-eat, and if you combine acid fruits with the whole-wheat bread, you will find usually that your trouble will almost immediately disappear, provided, of course, you take the exercises advised regularly.

EFFECTIVE MEANS OF CURE.

If, however, this does not bring relief, there are more effective means still that can be adopted to force the desired results. The massage or kneading process is a valuable assistant when all other means fail. Lie on the back. Now put a little sweet oil in the open hands, then bring them over the abdo-

men in all directions, pressing down vigorously. After continuing this for from three to
five minutes, roll the closed hand back and
forth over the abdomen, pressing vigorously
downward. In this part of the treatment
the hand should travel in a circle around the
abdomen. Beginning at the lower right
hand side, then go upward on right side,
over to upper left side, down left side to
lower left side, then over to lower right
side. This last kneading process, round and
round the abdomen, should be continued
from ten to fifteen minutes if case is at all
serious. It should be productive of satisfactory results, though after waiting a reason-
able time, you can then resort to the internal
bath treatment; that is, flushing the colon.
This will, of course, produce the desired
action, but it is well to avoid the use of this
means if possible as the bowels should not be
taught to depend on this unnatural means
for elimination. It is, however, so much
superior, so much more effective, than purga-
tives that there is no comparison. Purga-
tives cause serious injury, while this means
of emptying the bowels produces no evil

results. The only objection is that should its use be continued for a long period, the bowels would lose tone, and actually depend upon this means for an action.

Chapter XXV.

ABBREVIATED GENERAL INSTRUCTION FOR BUILDING NERVOUS AND SEXUAL POWER.

Rise when your desire for sleep has been satisfied.

Take the exercises prescribed nude, while reclining on your bed.

Follow these exercises with a friction bath

Then take a cold sitz and a sponge bath.

If you eat three meals per day, make your breakfast very light, preferably of fruits.

If your last meal is hearty, eat it as early as possible.

Sometime during the day take a long walk, with many deep breathing exercises.

Don't hurry!

Don't worry!

Take the special course of exercises just

before retiring after becoming inured to the work.

Don't cover too heavily when in bed.

Open the windows wide.

If you are a married man, occupy a bed by yourself.

Retire early enough to allow yourself eight hours of sleep.

Chapter XXVI.

DISEASES OF MEN.

It was not originally intended that the above subject should be treated here.

While writing on this book a young man called who had been inoculated with syphilitic poison about eight years previous. He had been treated with mercury by the highest authority on the medical board in one of our large Western cities. He supposed, of course, that such an eminent person would understand fully how to treat his trouble. He stated that, again and again in answer to his anxious inquiries, this physician assured him that the mercury in his system could easily be removed at any time, yet that after two years of the treatment, he began to make endeavors to remove the mercury from his system, but in vain. For six years he continued these endeavors, and had secured no relief; and the terrible tortures of mercurial poison.

ing that he described could not be fittingly depicted, and he stated that he would .rather be inoculated with syphilis a thousand times than to have the smallest drop of mercury in his system.

The experience of this young man, together with the influence of the other facts easily obtainable, caused the writer to fully realize the serious necessity for some practical knowledge of these subjects.

It has always been maintained that those who acquire such complaints fully deserve all they suffer. The writer does not hold such a belief. There are many who acquire the disease innocently, and even those with a guilty conscience only deserve to suffer according to the penalties made by Nature. These diseases unquestionably entail great suffering, but it was never intended that they should cling to the victim month after month, year after year, and even on to the end of life itself. Nature made no such penalties as this. These awful penalties were made by medical science. They are being perpetrated to-day by this same so-called science, and the writer has added this subject that those in the grasp of these horrible diseases may have an opportunity to escape after they have served the sentence that Nature demands as a punishment for their sins.

He has no desire to belittle the loathsome character of these diseases. Nature made them bad enough, but medical science has made them produce the most horrible, the most revolting objects that the human eye ever rested upon.

Methods of cure by natural means for the various sexual diseases are here presented. The results are as sure, if these methods are followed, as the conclusion derived from a mathematical problem, for the means of cure advised are based on natural laws, and cannot fail.

That there may be no question as to the authority of the writer in prescribing means of curing these diseases, he has purposely quoted every symptom and method of cure from works of members of the medical profession who have been able to go beyond the rules and regulations of the standard authorities recognized in their medical schools.

Do not make the mistake of adopting only

a part of the means of cure suggested. This will simply be wasting your time. Either try the methods advised here as given, or else leave it alone altogether. Of course, in troubles of this character it is far better to consult a physician, if you can find one familiar with rational means of curing these diseases, but if you value your sexual and general physical powers, do not, under any circumstances, allow any one to drug you to death. Drugs are useful only for antiseptic purposes and as a germicide.

Keep these facts plainly in view.

Chapter XXVII.

GONORRHEA.

COMMENTS ON THIS DISEASE BY VARIOUS AUTHORITIES.

" What unspeakable misery is entailed by suppressing gonorrhea. If done by means of injections, it frequently causes stricture; and to what misery this condition leads is best known to the many thousand victims of perverse medical treatment who suffer from it. Furthermore, frightful ravages are made alike by syphilis, and the mercury prescribed for it. Syphilis is the result of excesses and uncleanness. It can be cured only by cleansing every fibre of the body. Drug physicians, by treating merely the effects of the sin, can accomplish nothing. Under a natural régime. impure desires would be impossible. It is pitiful to see how powerless the drug schools are against these forms of disease. Any portion or portions of the body may be de.

stroyed by either the one or the other at any period after the infection. And yet nothing is more simple, prompt and rapid than cur. ing radically both gonorrhea and syphilis by hygienic means."—*A. F. Reinhold. Ph.D., M.D.*

Dr. H. N. Guernsey, in his excellent little book, "Plain Talks on Avoided Subjects," says: "When gonorrhea is contracted, although frequently suppressed by local treatment in the form of injections, it is never perfectly cured thereby. No; the hidden poison runs on for a lifetime, producing strictures, gleet and kindred diseases; finally, in old men, a horrible prostatis results, from which the balance of one's life is rendered miserable, indeed. If inflammation of the lungs supervenes, there is often a transmission of the virus to these vital organs, causing what is termed 'plastic pneumonia,' where one lobule after another becomes gradually sealed up, till nearly the whole of both lungs become impervious to air, and death results from asphyxia."

"The causes of gonorrhea, in the male, are produced from having intercourse with a woman having this disease, or from a woman having simply inflammation of the uterus, 'whites,' dysmenorrhea, or even if intercourse be had during the menstrual period. When produced in this last way, the man and woman—or husband and wife, as sometimes happens—must otherwise lead irregular and unhygenic lives; but established and reliable authorities have asserted that it may arise from intercourse with women who themselves have not the disease."—*John Cowan, M.D.*

In his book entitled "Transmission of Life," Dr. George H. Napheys, in speaking of this disease, says: "It may bring about life-long suffering, The passage from the bladder becomes inflamed and contracted. That organ itself is very apt to partake of the inflammation, and become irritable and sensitive. Spermatorrhea and impotence, with all their misery, may follow, and the whole economy may partake of the infection. An eruption of the skin, and an obstinate form of rheumatism, both wholly intractable to ordinary remedies, are more common than even many physicians imagine. Not infrequently these troublesome chronic, rheumatic complaints which annoy men in middle and advanced life are the late castigations which nature is inflicting for early transgressions.

"Medical records and journals are generally agreed that it is possible for pure and unoffending married people to suffer from an affection which closely resembles gonorrhea. This is caused by an acrid discharge from the female parts, or may be developed at the time of the monthly sickness of the wife. Physicians of unquestioned ability and honor declare this to be a fact, and assert that it is important that this should be known, as ignorance of this fact has led to unjust suspicions and cruel accusations, resulting in the disruption of families and the suffering of untold misery."—*Sylvanus Stall, D.D.*

SYMPTOMS OF THE DISEASE.

Dr. Druitt observes: "The patient first experiences a little itching or tingling at the orifice of the urethra, together with a sense of heat and soreness along the underside of the penis, and slight pain and scalding in making water. A little discharge soon exudes from the urethra; at first it is thin and whitish, but it soon becomes thick and puriform; and when the disease is at its height it is yellow or greenish, or tinged with blood. The penis swells, the gland is of a peculiar cherry color, is intensely tender, and often excoriated. In consequence of this tumefied state of the urethra, the stream of urine is small and forked, and passed with much straining and with severe pain. In addition to these symptoms there occur, in some cases, long-continued and painful erections, constituting chordee, or a highly painful and crooked state of the private member."

"The symptoms, appearing between the second and fifth day, are at first slight, there being an uneasy, tickling and smarting sensation at the mouth of the canal, which, on examination, is found to be more florid than usual, and moistened with a small quantity of colorless and viscid fluid, which glues the lips of the meatus together. This moisture, after a time, loses its clear, watery appearance, and assumes a milky hue. These early symptoms are present when the contagion is yet confined to the extreme portion of the urethra. This first stage generally lasts from

two to four days, when the symptons gradually become more intense, until, in about a
week after exposure, the second or inflammatory stage may be said to commence.
During this stage the mucus membrane
covering the glands has a reddened and angry
look, the extremity of the organ is swollen,
the discharge—now of a thick, yellowish,
creamy color—has become copious, there is
intense pain in passing the urine, excited by
the irritation produced by the salts contained
in the urine, and in consequence of the
urethra being contracted and more or less
obstructed by the discharge the stream is
forked, or otherwise irregular. A person
with gonorrhea is apt to be troubled with
nocturnal erections, when it often happens
that the penis is bent in the form of an arc,
producing chordee, caused by the effused
lymph on the under-surface of the organ
rendering it less extensible than the remaining portion. It sometimes happens that sym-
pathetically there is enlargment and tenderness of one or more glands in the groin, producing buboes. This second stage lasts from
one to three weeks. This is followed by the

third or final stage, which is characterized
only by the disappearance of the more prominent symptoms, and a gradual return to
health, the discharge becoming less and less
purulent, and finally completely disappear-
ing. This last stage may last for weeks or
months, depending on whether it is treated
and the mode of treating it."—*John Cowan,
M. D.*

METHODS OF TREATMENT.

"In the treatment of gonorrhea, the indications are first to restore the general health;
and second to allay the local inflammation.
It is a fact that cannot be gainsaid, that the
men who acquire such diseases are almost
invariably gross, as well as licentious, in
their habits of living. The first requirement
in the direction of a cure (and this will apply
with equal force to all acute diseases of the
sexual organs) is that the patient give up
the use of tobacco, alcoholic liquors, milk,
flesh, grease, seasoning and a stimulating
diet. He should live on the very plainest of
food, such as baked apples and potatoes, thin
gruel, unleavened bread. tomatoes, prunes,

oranges, etc. During the stage of acute inflammation, but very little of any kind of food should be taken; perfect rest, in a bed or on a lounge, should be observed. Next in importance to a right diet is bathing the whole body with tepid water, this to be repeated until the superficial heat is reduced to a normal standard. For the local treatment, sitz baths of tepid or cool water, varying in time from fifteen minutes to an hour— changing the water, if necessary—will afford decided relief. The sitz bath should be repeated as often as the inflammatory symptoms are aggravated. When resting, the genital parts should be enveloped in wet cloths.

The adoption of the above mode of treatment will effect a prompt and permanent cure, when a drug treatment, with its calomel, sugar of lead, caustic, copabia, cubebs, turpentine, etc., will not only aggravate the disease, but perhaps produce gleet, buboes or stricture."—*John Cowan, M.D.*

"Gonorrhea is in the beginning an inflammatory disease, and for this reason should be treated actively. The cooling wet compress upon the part affected, and the sitting bath, have great power over the disease; but it cannot be cut short speedily in all cases. It must, in fact, have a sort of course of its own; still a great deal may be done in mitigating its violence, and consequently in shortening its duration. The general treatment may be considered the same as for syphilis. The patient should be very careful not to overheat his blood, become too much frightened, or stand too long on the feet at a time. Do what we will, such cases sometimes run on for months; but gleet, so far as I am aware, does not follow this disorder when water (natural) . treatment is practiced.

It may be of interest to some to learn that there is no drug specific for this disease. If a medicine ever does any good under such circumstances, it is because of its effects on the constitution generally, and not of any direct power it may have over it. But drugging is a poor policy, making the best of it, and generally leaves the patient only the worse."—*Joel Shaw, M.D.*

You will note that the above methods of

treatment suppresses the disease; first, by thinning the blood and by removing all impurities from it with a very low diet; second, by assisting towards the elimination of impurities through the pores of the entire body with many baths each day; third, by sitz baths and by wet cloths applied to the organ itself, day and night if possible, the inflammation is allayed and much of the poison that is discharged ordinarily in pus through the urethra is taken up and discharged through the pores.

Thus the disease is actually hurried through its regular course, and complete recovery, with no possible after-results, is soon reached.

If so occupied that the advice of these physicians cannot be closely followed, here is practically the same treatment modified to suit a busy man's needs:

A friction bath immediately upon rising. (See chapter on Bathing.)

Follow immediately by a cold sitz bath. (See chapter on Bathing for description of a sitz bath.) Stay in this water from five to thirty minutes, as long as you can, and recu-

perate with a feeling of warmth. Before
rising from the bath wet the skin all over
and put on *underclothing at once without drying
the skin.*

Secure a heavy pair of trunks that you can
wear next the skin, something like very
short swimming trunks. Inside these trunks
you should wrap cloths wet in salted water
around the scrotum and the affected organ,
and wear this all day while at work, re-wet-
ting cloths whenever necessary.

It is far better to eat no breakfast, though
if you must eat, confine diet to appetizing
fruits.

Keep as quiet as you can during the day.

Eat lightly as possible at all meals. In
fact, the less you eat, the quicker recovery
can be expected.

Take cold sitz bath, same as in the morning, again before retiring. Put on night
clothes without drying the skin, and arrange
some way to keep the scrotum and affected
organ swathed in cloths wet with water, in
which some salt has been placed, during the
entire night.

If you must use an injection, have a physician or druggist subscribe a very *mild* solu-

tion of sulphate of zinc or of permanganate of potash. Though it may take longer to recover without the aid of these drugs, you will be better off in the end if they are not used.

CHAPTER XXVIII.

—

GLEET.

—

COMMENTS ON THE DISEASE.

"Gleet is an old or chronic discharge, arising from badly treated or neglected gonorrhea. It is often a troublesome matter, and many who have it are impotent besides, low-spirited, and desirous of making away with themselves. It is a singular fact that men who become bankrupt in this part of their organism, are apt to be tormented with suicidal propensities."—*Joel Shaw, M.D.*

"Gleet. When an attack of gonorrhea is badly treated, and not thoroughly cured, there may follow immediately, or perhaps not until after an interval of several weeks, or even months, a thin, watery discharge from the urethra, which is termed gleet. This discharge may continue for months, and in many cases, for years. In most cases of gleet the discharge is the only symptom. In some instances, however, there may be a feeling of uneasiness in the organ or peritoneum, or an itching about the glands, which may either be constant or attendant only upon the passage of the urine. In some cases the discharge is constant, and sufficiently copious to stain the linen, but in the majority it is perceptible only in the morning on rising. It is a well-established fact, that persons infected with gleet will communicate gonorrhea to healthy subjects, and that by aggravation gleet is readily transformed into gonorrhea. A hearty meal, alcoholic stimulants, sexual indulgence, violent exercise, exposure to sudden changes of temperature, may bring on a copious purulent discharge, attended by tumefaction of the parts, scalding in urination, and all the symptoms of acute gonorrhea."—*John Cowan, M. D.*

TREATMENT ADVISED.

"Gleet is to be managed on general principles; the system is to be purified and invigorated by baths, diet, etc., and the private member is to be kept constantly swathed in wet cloths. In all of these cases vegetarian diet is of great importance."—*Joel Shaw, M. D.*

"In the treatment of gleet the directions for general treatment in gonorrhea should be adopted. For the local treatment the sitz bath is indicated. Commencing with tepid water, which will slightly increase the discharge at first, the temperature should be daily lowered, so that at the end of a week very cold water may be used. This bath may be applied two or three times a day, fifteen to twenty minutes at a time. The case of a gentleman who had gleet at this moment occurs to me. It had been of some two years' duration, the patient having tried the best physicians in vain. Drugs, applications and injections of all kinds had been tried, only to make the discharge seem worse. The patient had the offer of a sea trip on a sailing vessel, which he accepted. The trip lasted for nearly three months, during which time, owing to peculiar circumstances, the food was not only of the plainest in quality, but of the smallest in quantity. The patient landed in better health than he had for a long time experienced, and entirely cured of his gleet. I mention this case simply to show that in this disease, as in almost all others of a sexual nature, if the patient would adopt a line of life involving in it pure air and plenty of it, simple diet and little of it, rest, cleanliness of body, freedom from tobacco, alcoholic liquors and sexual intercourse, it would absolutely be all that would be required to cure him of his disease and restore him to perfect health."—*John Cowan, M.D.*

You will note that the principal difference in the treatment of gonorrhea and gleet is that in the treatment of gleet, abundance of exercise is advised, while in acute gonorrhea no more exercise should be taken than is absolutely necessary. If gonorrhea becomes chronic, however, it should be treated the same as gleet.

CHAPTER XXIX

STRICTURE OF THE URETHRA.

COMMENTS ON STRICTURE.

"Strictures of the urethra may be classified as transitory or permanent—transitory when the result of muscular spasm, congestion or inflammation—permanent, when through wrong treatment of the urethral canal. Transitory stricture of the inflammatory form is produced by gonorrhea and its maltreatment, and the injudicious use of catheters or bougies. It is known by local heat, pain or swelling, with inability to urinate, unless with extreme pain. When of the spasmodic variety, it is usually seated at the neck of the bladder. It may be induced by violent exercise, long retention of the urine, or sexual excesses. Permanent stricture may be located in any part of the urethra, but it more frequently occurs in the membraneous and bulbous portions of the canal. It generally comes on slowly and insidiously. The individual first observes a few drops of water remain after the whole seems to have been discharged, then notices a fine spiral or divided stream, and lastly, discharges his urine by drops only, requiring a long time to empty the bladder. It occasionally happens that the patient loses all control, and the urine dribbles away continually."—*John Cowan, M. D.*

METHODS OF TREATMENT ADVISED.

"The usual methods in treating stricture are by the introduction of bougies, the application of caustic, or by incision—all impossible in the home treatment of the disease. If the patient will but firmly resolve to lead a rigidly plain and simple life—absolute freedom from all stimulating food and drink, tobacco, flesh meat, etc., eating less of plain food than the system is capable of assimilating, living a strictly continent life, and, along with the every-day general bath, to take twice a day, for half an hour at a time, a cool or cold water sitz bath, drinking nothing but pure water, and as much of it as may be desired, he will, in the course of from one to three months, be thoroughly cured of transitory stricture, and in from four to twelve months—depending much on the previous habits of the individual—he will be cured of permanent stricture, and that without any of the dangers of after-results attendant on the introduction of bougies, caustic, etc. The very worst cases of permanent stricture, after long trials and failures with bougies, etc., have in this way been permanently removed and effectually cured."—*John Cowan, M.D.*

"Stricture is sometimes a result of gonorrhea, as well as of syphilis, and may often be relieved by the cold compress, the cold sitting bath, the cold general bath, wet sheet pack, etc. The sooner it is treated, the better the prospect of a cure without surgical operation. A thorough course of hunger (fasting) cure is excellent in cases of this kind."—*Joel Shaw, M.D.*

CHAPTER XXX.

CHANCROID (SOMETIMES CALLED SOFT CHANCRE.)

COMMENTS ON THIS DISEASE BY DIFFERENT AUTHORITIES.

"A chancroid is a painful ulcer or sore, which secretes a contagious matter, usually appearing upon the genitals within a few days after exposure. If not properly treated, these sores often last several months. There may be several present at the same time. In many cases, a painful swelling occurs in the groin, or on one side or on both, from enlagement of the glands in this region. The swelling may disappear by absorption, or suppurate and form an abscess. This form of veneral disease does not give rise to constitutional symptoms."—*A. A. Kellogg, M.D.*

The following are the symptoms of a chancroid when fully formed:

"Its outline is circular, unless modified by the shape of the solution of continuity in which it is implanted; it has a punched-out appearance; the edges are jagged, abrupt and sharply cut, and do not adhere closely to the subadjacent tissues; the fluid secretion is copious and purulent, and it is surrounded by an areola which varies in width and depth of color with the degree of inflammation present. They are more frequently multiple than single; but when one chancroid appears at the outset as the immediate result of contagion, others are apt to spring up around it from successive inoculation, since the original ulcer pours out an abundant secretion, and its presence confers no immunity against others."

In the comparison of the three poisons of gonorrhea, the chancroid and syphilis, Bumstead, in his "Venereal Diseases," says:

"The only property common to them all is their communication, for the most part, by contact with the genital or gans. The poisons of gonorrhea and of the chancroid are alike, in that their action is limited and *never extends to the general system:* nor does one attack afford the slightest protection against a second. They differ in that the poison of gonorrhea may arise spontaneously, while that of chancroid, so far as we know, never thus originates; that gonorrhea, chiefly affects the surface—true ulceration being rarely induced—and, in its complications, most frequently attacks parts connected with the original seat of the disease by a continuous mucus surface, as the prostate gland, bladder and testicles; while the chancroid, on the contrary, is an ulcer involving the whole thickness of the integument or mucous membrane, and its complications are seated in the absorbent vessels and ganglia. It would also appear that the poisons of these two affections are limited to one common vehicle—namely, pus. This conclusion is sustained by the fact that neither the poison of gonorrhea nor that of the chancroid ever reaches the general circulation, and it is well known that pus globules are not capable of absorption. When the purulent matter of a chancroid enters the absorbent vessels, as occurs in the formatism of a virulent bubo, it is arrested by the first chain of lymphatic ganglia and goes no further. The syphilitic virus is alone capable of infecting the system at large, and of affording protection by its presence against subsequent attacks. Unlike the poisons of gonorrhea and the chancroid, it is not limited to purulent matter, but exists in the blood, in the fluids of the secondary lesions, in the semen, and probably in other secretions. There is no opposition whatever between these three poisons; they may all coexist in the same person, who may at the same time have gonorrhea, a chancroid, and a chancre of the syphilitic lesion."

"The chancroid arises only in consequence of contagion from its like. It is most generally found in the vicinity of the genital organs, although it is sometimes found in urethra, vagina and rectum, or wherever there is a mucous surface. It is rarely met on the head or face, where, on the contrary, the initial lesion of syphilis is not uncommon. The vehicle of the chancroid virus is the secretion of the ulcer, which, if it be inserted beneath the epidermis of any other part of the body, a chancroid is equally the result." —*John Cowan, M.D.*

TREATMENT ADVISED.

" Treatment.— Keep the sore clean, employ a restricted diet, practice absolute continence, and refrain from active exercise for a few days. Meat, stimulants, spices and tobacco should be carefully avoided. The specific poison may be destroyed by touching the sore with a strong caustic of some sort."— *A. A. Kellogg, M.D.*

"In the treatment of chancroid, prompt attention to the general health of the individ. ual is almost all that is required, for the disease, being a self-limited one, it will get well in the absence of all treatment, *other than that of perfect cleanliness of the parts.* But when not promptly attended to by the adop- tion of a strict diet of plain food and bathing it is apt to be followed by a bubo. If the pustule is noticed the second or third day after contagion, it can be destroyed by burn- ing with nitrate of silver; but after this time —say, within from three to six days—nitrate of silver will be too feeble, and it will require the application of a much more powerful caustic, as nitric of sulphuric acid, applied by means of a glass rod with a rounded extrem.

ity, although a simple piece of wood—an ordinary lucifer match—will do. On the acid first touching the ulcer, the pain for an instant will be very severe, but it becomes much less acute on subsequent applications, of which there should be several to render the destruction complete. Great care must be taken to prevent the acid from touching the neighboring surfaces, which should be protected by dry lint or other material. When it is too late to apply the acid, cloths wet in water should be kept on the parts affected, and often changed. When the application of acid has produced suppuration, the wet (linen) cloths should also be employed. This, with the perfect cleanliness of the parts, and perfect cleanliness of the cloths used, and careful attention to the general health. will always result in a cure."
—*John Cowan, M.D.*

A physician of long experience with these diseases informed the writer that if a piece of absorbent cotton, wet in " Black Wash," which any druggist or physician can prescribe, is kept on the sore continually, night and day, the disease germ will be destroyed and the sore healed in but a short time, *provided the habits of life are strictly in conformity to the ordinary laws of hygiene and health.* If the sore is under the foreskin of the organ this can easily be done. Merely draw the foreskin back, place the piece of wet cotton on the sore, and then draw the foreskin down over the cotton, Place fresh pieces of wet cotton on the sore night and morning. If the sore appears where this cannot be .done, other means will have to be devised to hold the wet cotton on the sore.

The above mentioned drug will be found far safer and surer to use in combination with the hygienic treatment than those prescribed by Dr. Cowan, though the reader can take his choice.

Chapter XXXI.

BUBOES.

COMMENTS ON THE DISEASE.

Bumstead divides buboes into three classes: First; the simple, inflammatory bubo, the symptoms of which are a swelling in the groin, attended with tenderness on pressure and pain, which is aggravated by pressure or the standing posture. The gland is felt to be somewhat enlarged, but is still movable beneath the integument, which preserves its normal color. This condition may last for an indefinite period, during the continuation of the ulcer, or even after its cicatrization, and yet finally disappear without suppuration. In simple inflammatory bubo, most frequently, only one gland is affected; if others are involved, they are commonly so to a less degree. In less fortunate cases, the inflammatory symptoms increase in severity;

the tumor acquires larger dimensions, and becomes adherent to the skin and underlying fascia, so that it is no longer movable; the pain and tenderness are increased; motion is difficult; the skin becomes reddened; suppuration is ushered in with a chill; the presence of matter is indicated by a soft spot in the midst of the general hardness, and soon after by distinct fluctuation; and although resolution is still possible, yet commonly the contents of the abscess are discharged through an opening in the integument formed by the process of ulceration.

Second; the virulent bubo, which receives its names from the fact that the pus which it contains is contagious, and will upon artificial inoculation give rise to a chancroid. A virulent bubo is due to the absorption of virus from the surface of a chancroid, and its conveyance, by means of the lymphatics, to the ganglion. It is usually situated on the same side as the chancroid, but sometimes upon the opposite side, and sometimes both groins are effected, especially when the ulcer is upon any part in the median line. Prior to its spontaneous or artificial opening, the course of a virulent bubo is that of a simple bubo, and the patient should understand that the early symptoms of the two are identical; though the distinction between them is fully justified by the inevitable suppuration and specific properties of the one, and the possible resolution and simple character of the other.

Third; the indolent bubo, the inflammation of which is of a subacute character, closely resembling the well-known scrofulous inflammation of the glands of the neck in children. There may be a moderate amount of pain, tenderness on pressure, and difficulty of motion, although these are rarely severe or of long continuance. The tumor very slowly enlarges, perhaps to the size of a hen's egg; the skin covering it becomes thin, and of a livid red color, and fluctuation can be detected without being ushered in by chills and fevers, as in the case of inflammatory bubo. After a time several openings form spontaneously, and there escapes a thin, flaky, watery-looking fluid.

" Buboes. This is an affection of the lymphatic ganglion, dependent, in the great majority of cases, upon the presence of a chancroid, although they may be caused by gonorrhea or sexual excess. A bubo, with a primary syphilitic sore, or chancre, which is accompanied by induration of the ganglia, which never suppurates unless under the influence of some additional exciting cause. The occurrence of buboes is favored by a scrofulous constitution, by wrongly-treated chancroids, by mechanical violence, undue exercise, excesses in diet, and by sexual intercourse during the existence of a chancroid or gonorrhea."—*John Cowan, M.D.*

TREATMENT ADVISED FOR THIS DISEASE.

" The existence of buboes usually indicate the presence of a soft or hard chancre or chancres, and immediate means should be adopted to destroy the disease germs in these sores. The buboes will usually begin to disappear when this is done."

"The object to be aimed at in the treatment of buboes is to subdue inflammation and avert suppuration, if possible. To this end, perfect rest and a low diet of plain, simple food, is of the first importance. In the early stages, cold wet cloths, frequently renewed, should be constantly kept on the swelling. Three or four times a day the parts may be fomented for fifteen or twenty minutes at a time, and then immediately after covered with cold wet cloths, over which dry ones should be placed. Twice a day a sitz bath, moderately cool, may be employed. The close observance of these rules in the early stages will certainly prevent suppuration; but should the bubo indicate by its tenseness and throbbing pain the commencement of suppuration, warm wet cloths should be constantly employed until matter forms, when, if the abscess does not open spontaneously, it should be cut with a lancet."—*John Cowan, M. D.*

CHAPTER XXXII.

SYPHILIS.

COMMENTS ON HOW THIS DREADED DISEASE IS ACQUIRED, AND OTHER INFORMATION IN REFERENCE TO IT BY VARIOUS AUTHORITIES.

"Syphilis is more frequently communicated by impure coition, although there are various other ways of acquiring the disease. It has been sometimes caught by sucking the nipple of an infected wet nurse; by infected saliva communicated in the act of kissing; by drinking out of a cup that had previously been used by a syphilitic patient; by lying in a bed which had been antecedently occupied by a person laboring under the disease; by being bled with an infected lancet; by being shaved with an infected razor; by the attendance of an infected midwife, and the disease is said even to have communicated through the breath of one tainted with the malady."—*Joel Shaw, M.D.*

"Syphilis is propagated in various ways, but in most cases it depends principally upon sexual intercourse. Being an infectious disease, the presence of the virus, when brought in contact with surfaces covered with thin epidermis, or when denuded of its cuticle, it is transmitted from one individual to another."—*John Cowan, M. D.*

Dr. Napheys, in speaking of the ulcer which form in the mouth, says: "The discharge from them is a poison, and can convey the disease, and so can a drop of blood from the infected person."

Dr. Hollick also says: "It is not positively known whether the semen itself from a man who has syphilis will give it to the woman with whom he cohabits. That is, suppose he contracts syphilis and is cured so far that there is no sore from which the woman can be infected, may she be so from the semen? There is good reason to suppose she may, in the same way that she would be from the man's blood." The same author also says: "Most usually the child inherits syphilis from its mother, who may contract it from the father without being aware of what is the matter. But the child may also be affected from the father through the semen, which may, undoubtedly, be contaminated by syphilis. In all probability the disease affects the seminal animalculæ, making them feeble and imperfect, so that if they impregnate, the resulting offspring will be feeble and imperfect also. Probably this is one reason why women, when impregnated by syphilitic men, are so apt to miscarry. The embryo has not life enough to retain itself in the womb. Through how many generations syphilis may run before it becomes extinct we do not know, but with each remove it seems to become more modified and lighter, till at last it probably merges into some ordinary form of disease, especially scrofula."

Dr. Hollick says: "The father may be so far well that he will not disease the mother by connection, but he will beget a child diseased through the semen, and this child will infect its own mother before its birth."

The same author says: "The poison by syphilis does not reside in the sores only, but infects the blood of the patient. If blood be taken from the man who has syphilis, and inoculated into another man, it will give him syphilis, the same as if he had been inoculated with matter from the chancre."

Upon the subject of inspection and protection, Dr. Guernsey, in "Plain Talks," says: "There is no safety among impure or loose women, whether in private homes or in the very best regulated houses of illfame; even in Paris, where, after women have been carefully examined and pronounced free from any infecting condition, the first man who visits one of them often carried away a deadly enemy in his blood which had lurked in concealment beyond the keen eye of the inspector. A young man, or a man at any age, is in far greater danger amidst company of this stamp than he would be with a clear conscience and pure character in the midst of the wildest forest full of all manner of poisonous serpents and wild beasts of every description. A knowledge of the above facts should be enough to chill the first impulse and to make any man who respects his own well-being turn away and flee from the destruction that awaits him."

An intelligent physician, who has given much time and study to the consideration of this subject, in writing says: "In the great cities it is fearfully prevalent, including both sexes and all grades of society. We do not doubt that more than 25 per cent. of the whole population is more or less tainted with it, and the greater number innocently. Nor is it at all confined to the indigent and degraded. It holds just as firm, though concealed and held in check, in the fashionable clubs and stately mansions of the opulent as in the alleys and back slums of the dregs of our population. No man, no woman, we care not what his or her position or his or her life may be, is secure from its loathsome touch."

SCATHING CONDEMNATIONS OF THE MERCURY TREATMENT.

Dr. Bennett says that "more than eighty thousand cases have been submitted to experiment, by means of which it has been perfectly established that syphilis is cured in a shorter time, and with less probability of producing secondary syphilis, by the simple than by the mercurial method." The same author further remarks: "The intensity of the disease in modern times has declined exactly in proportion as its treatment by mercury has diminished, and the disorder been left to follow its natural course."

"For a long time it was believed that mercury is a specific for the syphilitic poison; but the notion is not at the present time held by any respectable authority. It is admitted, moreover, that the horrible symptoms of secondary syphilis have in many instances been, to say the least, greatly aggravated by this drug."—*Joel Shaw, M. D.*

It is the opinion of many that a few doses of mercury, in some one of its many forms, will cure syphilis. This is a great error. Mercury, nor no other drug, has ever cured, or ever will cure, syphilis—or, for that matter, any other disease. The use of mercury in this disease, instead of curing it, simply for a time prevents its outward manifestation, and when the peculiar effect of the mercurial poison has weakened, the syphilitic poison—more virulent and more destructive than ever—again appears, making it more difficult than ever for the life-force of the individual to get rid of it. Allowing two persons to have syphilis, one of them to be treated with mercury, and the other without mercury, or any treatment whatever, I would in the end much rather be the possessor of the constitution of the individual who had used no mercury or other treatment than that of the one who had used mercury." —*John Cowan, M. D.*

"The effect of mercury, in syphilis, was measured at one time," says Dr. Dunglison, "by the amount of saliva discharged. If the disease were of a certain duration, the patient must spit a quart; if of longer, two quarts, and so on; but now, since the conviction of the practioner is, that salivation is rarely ever necessary, and that it is rather to be deplored—inasmuch as the increasing discharge exhausts and irritates, without being of itself beneficial—the practice has been abandoned; and if we meet with excessive ptyalism, it is generally in those who are easily affected by mercury, and in whom the affection supervenes rapidly, or in those whom the remedy has by accident been persisted in for a longer period than was contemplated.   The books were formerly filled with descriptions of the horrible accidents induced by mercurial ptyalism, some of which the author has witnessed, an excessive sloughing, loss of teeth, caries of jaw-bones, protrusion of the tongue from the mouth, adhesions of the lips and cheeks, etc., with at times excessive febrile action, marasmus, and death."

CHAPTER XXXIII.

CAN SYPHILIS BE ENTIRELY CURED?

SHOULD TAINTED PERSONS MARRY?

"There is a great difference of opinion among physicians concerning the treatment and the curability of this disease. The eminent Prof. Van Buren, of New York, who has had a very extensive experience in the treatment of this affection, stated in our hearing, a few years ago, that he never dared to assure a patient that he was well, no matter how completely free from disease he might seem to be. Others claim to be able to affect a cure in nearly all cases. Mercury has been looked upon as the great antidote for syphilis; but there are grounds for doubting the efficacy of this drug."—*A. A. Kellog, M. D.*

Dr. Guernsey, the author of "Plain Talks on Avoided Subjects," may be regarded as a fair sample of those who believe that the disease can be thoroughly eradicated. In his book he says: " An experience of nearly forty years of the treatment of these cases in both sexes, has given me the power to know whereof I speak; and I do declare that a very large percentage of these cases can be cured in a safe manner, and so perfectly cured, too, that there will be no danger of transmitting the infection to the offspring. I by no means stand alone in this statement; many other physicians, after long years of experience, assert the same truth."

" We once had a patient who, sixteen years before, had contracted syphilis. He was un-lucky enough to try first the drug schools, which treated him with mercury during all those years, and of course unsuccessfully. At the time of his application to us, he had large clusters of gummy tumors in three parts of his body. When told that plain water would cure him, he hesitated to rely on water alone, as he could not understand how water could have the power to cure, where mercury had for sixteen long years failed. We cannot blame him, when medical men also fail to understand this simple truth. Considerable persuasion was required to induce him to give up the use of the mercury; but we eventually succeeded, and after a treatment of two months the man was cured. Our system of cleansing, first softened the gummy tumors; then blood and pus passed away; and finally the tumors grew more and more shallow, until they entirely closed up."—*A. F. Reinhold, Ph. D., M. D.*

" It is sometimes asked, in the case of persons who have had syphilis, how soon could they marry, without the chance of entailing the disease on their offspring, and it is a question rather difficult to decide. If the disease has not yet passed into the constitutional stage, and the reform plan of treatment here given be adopted and faithfully observed for two years, I think the system of a naturally strong person would in this time be entirely free from the taint of syphilis. If the disease has passed into the constitutional stage, and has in a measure destroyed parts of the body by ulceration, it may require for its total extinction the close and faithful observance of hygienic and reform remedial measures for from five to eight years, and even then there might be doubts of its non-transmissibility."—*John Cowan, M. D.*

"The drug schools in comparing gonorrhea and syphilis consider the latter the more serious of the two. They apply injections and internal drugs for gonorrhea, and local caustics and mercury for syphilis. Under the drug system, both forms of disease may be followed by the most terrible consequences. Syphilis, especially, is never radically cured by drugs. By our natural methods we can absolutely and thoroughly cure fresh cases of either disease in a few days, and old cases in a few months."—*A. F. Reinhold, Ph.D., M.D.*

SYMPTOMS AND COMPLETE DESCRIPTION OF THE DISEASE BY VARIOUS AUTHORITIES.

"The primary stage is recognized by the appearance of the indurated or hard chancre, or ulcer, which usually begins as a pimple, and after several days develops into an inflamed, open ulcer or chancre, having a red circle. These sores may be attended by the swelled groin or buboes, and after a few weeks both may yield to treatment and disappear, but this is the source of no intelligent comfort, for the serious trouble has only begun.

"The secondary symptoms which follow, manifest themselves in a virulent attack of the disease upon the skin and mucous membrane. The secondary stage is reached at the end of a few weeks, usually three or four, or it may remain dormant for that many months. The attack now is upon the skin. Rashes, eruptions and sores appear upon the body. The glands inflame and gather. Shallow ulcers form upon the tongue and just back of the lips on the inside of the mouth. The throat ulcerates, catarrh lays hold of the mucous chambers of the head; the stomach, the liver, and the internal organs may be attacked. The hair is apt to loosen and fall out, the spirit becomes depressed, the brain may be involved, and imbecility, epilepsy and insanity may follow. These are some of the terrors and horrors of the secondary stage. The next is still worse.

"In the tertiary stage the disease leaves the outer surfaces and attacks the bones.

The early symptom is a severe pain like rheumatism, not at the joints, but between them, especially between the knee and the ankle and on the head. The pain is severe at night, and its victim often walks the floor, unable to lie down or sleep. The bones become brittle, and nature loses her power to heal. The nose is liable to be eaten away, and piece by piece, through great sores in the flesh, the bones slough and pass out, or they may weaken and break by a sudden strain."—*Sylvanus Stall, D.D.*

"Syphilis has three distinct stages. The first is a local manifestion, known as chancre. Two or three weeks, or longer, after exposure, a small, hard, reddish pimple makes its appearance, usually upon the genitals, although cases have occurred in which the disease was contracted by kissing, when the chancre was formed upon the lip. The pimple increases in size for a few days, and finally ulcerates, and discharges slightly. It does not usually give much inconvenience, and is, in fact, not infrequently unnoticed. In this respect the chancre differs much from the chancroid, a very important distinction-

After a few days the glands of the groins become somewhat enlarged, although not very painful. After one to three months the secondary stage of the disease appears, as an eruption of red spots, which are followed by pimples. After a time, larger pimples or pustules make their appearance, leaving behind them pock marks like those of small pox. Ulcers also appear in some cases. Simultaneously with the occurrence of the eruption, slightly raised spots of a whitish color, known as mucous patches, appear on the mucous membrane of the lips and tongue. A slight discharge arises from these patches, which is of a very contagious character. The patient also has sore throat, and often sore eyes, and after the general health has become considerably impaired, suffers greatly with pains in the head, arms, legs, breast, and particularly in the joints, though the pain is not confined to them as in rheumatism. Small swellings, known as nodes, which are tender on pressure, appear on the shins and other parts.

"The above symptoms disappear after a few weeks, and the patient may seem to be

well for several months or years; but unless
the disease has been properly treated, it is
all the time at work in the system, and next
makes its appearance in the deeper tissues,
particularly in the bones and cartilages of
the nose and skull. Not infrequently the
nose is greatly disfigured, or even wholly
destroyed. The liver, lungs, kidneys, heart
and other internal organs, are also likely to
be affected. No other disease makes such
fearful ravages in the human constitution as
this."—*A. A. Kellogg, M.D.*

SYMPTOMS.

"Symptoms.—These are of two kinds—the
primary and the secondary. The primary
symptoms consist of chancres, or ulcers,
appearing most frequently on the genitals
from the third to the tenth day after infection. These ulcers vary in character and
appearance, according to the individual's
constitution and the nature or virulence of
the poison from which they originate.
Bubo, or a painful swelling of the lymphatic
vessel or gland of the groin, is also one of
the primary symptoms of syphilis. In gen-

eral, the bubo ulcerates and breaks, and, in some cases, causes a tedious and troublesome sore.   It is a very painful affair.

"The secondary symptoms occur usually in five or six weeks after the primary; but sometimes earlier, and, in other instances, at a much later date—several months at least.   For sometime before their appearance, the patient is generally thin and wan; looks dispirited; his eyes are heavy; and he complains of want of sleep and of rheumatic pains.   The skin and mucous membrane of the throat are generally the parts first affected—the symptoms consisting of eruptions of an obstinate character, and ulcers, which, as well as the latter, take on a variety of forms and appearances.   The eyes are also very apt to become diseased; but the most horrible phase of the affection is that of the bones.   These often become extensively affected, and, indeed, as we may well say, rotten, causing an amount of suffering, more especially at night, which may well remind us of the fabled tortures of the damned."—*Joel Shaw, M. D.*

Chapter XXXIV.

TREATMENT ADVISED.

"The more rational principle of treatment—the one now adopted by the more intelligent among practitioners—is not to look upon medicines as a specific for syphilis, but to adopt such means as are best calculated for the good of the constitution generally.

"With regard to chancre, many are of opinion that if it can be removed at once on its appearance, the system is in great part saved from the venereal infection. It is customary to cauterize the sore as soon as it appears. Local wet compresses to the parts should be used unremittingly; the wet-sheet pack should, if possible, be used often, the diet should be strictly vegetable, and the whole management, both as regards the primary and the secondary symptoms, should be such as is best calculated to purify and invigorate the body generally. The hunger-fasting cure is nowhere more applicable."—*Joel Shaw, M. D.*

"According to Prof. Hughes Bennett, M. D., F. R. S. E., President of the Royal Medical Society of Edinburgh, the mercurial treatment is being rapidly superseded by the 'simple' method, which consists in careful regulation of all the habits of the patient, good hygiene, avoidence of spices, condiments, meat, and all stimulating foods, and the use of tepid baths and other eliminative treatment. Two or three full baths may be taken daily with advantage, unless the patient is very weak. The vapor, hotair, Turkish, and Russian baths are also useful. The wet-sheet pack is a very admirable remedy. Fomentations and tepid compresses should be applied to irritable parts. The patient should drink from one to two quarts of water daily. · By these means the poison may be eliminated from the system; while by the mercurial treatment, according to Dr. Bennett and several other eminent German physicians, the manifestation of the disease is only checked, thus merely delaying the expulsion of the poison from the system.

"In order to be effectual, the treatment must be continued for months after the symptoms of the disease have disappeared, as the malady may appear even after the lapse of many years, and if not in the lifetime of the transgressor, may appear in his posterity."—*A. A. Kellog, M. D.*

"In the first stages, immediately the nature of the sore has been decided to be a chancre, the patient should look to the conditions and regulate his general system. If he uses tobacco and alcoholic liquors, he must discard them completely. He should avoid all gross and stimulating food, and all manner of spices and condiments, as well as tea, coffee and chocolate. He should confine his diet to the smallest possible quantity of ripe fruits, bread made from unbolted wheat flour, cracked corn, cracked wheat, etc., and pure water. This may seem a rigid and severe initial requirement in the treatment, but as it is the only possible way of assisting Nature to throw off the poison, the patient must adopt it in full measure if a radical cure is earnestly desired. Next in importance to diet is bathing. Upon rising in the morning the patient should take a sitz bath, and at the same time a foot bath. The water in the sitz bath should be, at the commencement, of a tepid temperature, and gradually lowered until it is cold —as cold as the patient can comfortably bear it. The water of the foot bath should be warm, and increased in temperature until it becomes hot. At the close of the bath it should never be neglected to dash cold water on the feet, or dip them for a moment into cold water. This sitz and foot bath should last from 15 to 30 minutes. Between 10 and 11 o'clock A. M. this hip and foot bath should be repeated, followed by a general bath of the whole body, given thoroughly, effectually and rapidly. After drying, through friction of the whole body by the hand, from 5 to 15 minutes by the patient, and, if convenient, assisted by an assistant; this should on no account be neglected. Should the sun shine, allow its rays to fall directly on the patient's nude body during the time of friction. Before going to bed, which should be at an early hour in the evening, the sitz bath should be repeated, with the addition that, before it is taken, cloths wet in hot water should be wrapped around the loins, half way down the thighs, and including the generative organs. These should be kept on until there is decided redness of the skin after taking them off, to be immediately followed by the sitz bath, the water of which should be, as already mentioned, of a tepid temperature, and gradually increased during the bath to as low a temperature as the patient can bear and readily react after.

"Abundant exercise—when possible, in open air—should always be had.

"Great care must be employed in keeping surface sores perfectly clean, and all cloths, water, etc., used about them should be handled with great care, as the exuding virulent matter, even when diluted, is capable, when brought into contact with any *abraded* surface, of propagating the disease.

"To entirely free the system of the disease, it may be necessary to follow up

this line of treatment for years. Day after day, month after month, and year after year, the patient should never neglect to closely follow all the requirements necessary to the regaining of a clean, sweet, healthy body, free from the faintest syphilitic taint."
—*J. H. Cowan, M. D.*

You will note a general agreement in the advice of the three physicians here quoted. They practically concur as to the method of treatment. Each advocate means that will tend to build up the general health and cleanse the system of the poison.

For one occupied all day in some employment, the following regime would be about the same as prescribed and no doubt be more satisfactorily followed.

Five or ten minutes active exercise on rising, exercise to be followed by a thorough friction bath. Follow by a cold sitz bath. (See chapter on Bathing for description of sitz bath and Friction Bath.) Stay in the bath from 5 to 30 minutes. Exercise after coming out of the bath until warm before putting on underwear. After thoroughly warm dash water all over the body and put on underwear with skin wet.

If buboes and chancre have appeared, wear cloths all day wet in salted water, over them in a pair of trunks as described in treatment for gonorrhea. Change and rewet these cloths two or three times per day.

Eat as little as you possibly can and live. Avoid all meats.

Go without breakfast. Encourage appetite for fruit.

If inclined to be full blooded take a steam or hot-air bath every day or two.

Drink all the pure water you can without actual discomfort.

Do not fail to take a long walk, with many deep breathing exercises, sometime during the day.

If you could live on one very light meal per day, for a time, it will make beneficial results appear almost immediately. The less you eat the more quickly the taint can be permanently eliminated.

Take a cold sitz bath at night, same as in the morning, warming the body before and afterwards with exercise.

Arrange some wet cloths so they will remain in direct contact with the organs and the groin during the entire night. Wet a light blanket or a very heavy sheet in water, wring it out partially, then lay it on the bed and wrap it around your nude body immediately on retiring. Put sufficient cover over this for warmth and sleep thus until morning.

Be very careful to breathe pure air at all times. Follow this treatment accurately and you will find it will cleanse the body of the syphilitic taint sooner than any other possible means.

You must not expect to have the same amount of energy when following this treatment as is usual, for the constant drain on the pores in this continuous water treatment tends to lessen the feeling of energy. But your system is being cleansed and that is the only object one should have who happens to be tainted with this disease.

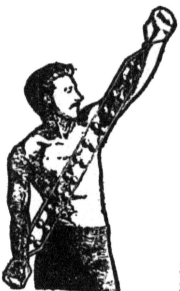
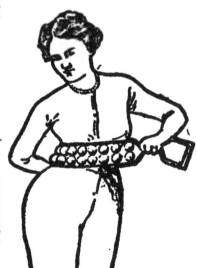

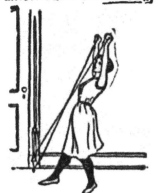
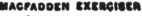
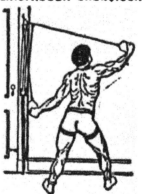

Made in the USA
Las Vegas, NV
20 December 2022

63620887R00138